T0227318

Peripheral Nerves: Injuries

Guest Editors

ROBERT J. SPINNER, MD
CHRISTOPHER J. WINFREE, MD

NEUROSURGERY
CLINICS OF NORTH AMERICA

www.neurosurgery.theclinics.com

Consulting Editors

ANDREW T. PARSA, MD, PhD
PAUL C. McCORMICK, MD, MPH

January 2009 • Volume 20 • Number 1

SAUNDERS an imprint of ELSEVIER, Inc.

W.B. SAUNDERS COMPANY
A Division of Elsevier Inc.

1600 John F. Kennedy Blvd. • Suite 1800 • Philadelphia, PA 19103-2899

http://www.theclinics.com

NEUROSURGERY CLINICS OF NORTH AMERICA Volume 20, Number 1
January 2009 ISSN 1042-3680, ISBN-13: 978-1-4377-0506-5, ISBN-10: 1-4377-0506-5

Editor: Joanne Husovski
Developmental Editor: Donald Mumford

© 2008 Elsevier ■ All rights reserved.

This journal and the individual contributions contained in it are protected under copyright by Elsevier, and the following terms and conditions apply to their use:

Photocopying
Single photocopies of single articles may be made for personal use as allowed by national copyright laws. Permission of the Publisher and payment of a fee is required for all other photocopying, including multiple or systematic copying, copying for advertising or promotional purposes, resale, and all forms of document delivery. Special rates are available for educational institutions that wish to make photocopies for non-profit educational classroom use. For information on how to seek permission visit www.elsevier.com/permissions or call: (+44) 1865 843830 (UK)/(+1) 215 239 3804 (USA).

Derivative Works
Subscribers may reproduce tables of contents or prepare lists of articles including abstracts for internal circulation within their institutions. Permission of the Publisher is required for resale or distribution outside the institution. Permission of the Publisher is required for all other derivative works, including compilations and translations (please consult www.elsevier.com/permissions).

Electronic Storage or Usage
Permission of the Publisher is required to store or use electronically any material contained in this journal, including any article or part of an article (please consult www.elsevier.com/permissions). Except as outlined above, no part of this publication may be reproduced, stored in a retrieval system or transmitted in any form or by any means, electronic, mechanical, photocopying, recording or otherwise, without prior written permission of the Publisher.

Notice
No responsibility is assumed by the Publisher for any injury and/or damage to persons or property as a matter of products liability, negligence or otherwise, or from any use or operation of any methods, products, instructions or ideas contained in the material herein. Because of rapid advances in the medical sciences, in particular, independent verification of diagnoses and drug dosages should be made.

Although all advertising material is expected to conform to ethical (medical) standards, inclusion in this publication does not constitute a guarantee or endorsement of the quality or value of such product or of the claims made of it by its manufacturer.

Neurosurgery Clinics of North America (ISSN 1042-3680) is published quarterly by Elsevier Inc., 360 Park Avenue South, New York, NY 10010-1710. Months of issue are January, April, July, and October. Business and Editorial Offices: 1600 John F. Kennedy Blvd., Suite 1800, Philadelphia, PA 19103-2899. Customer Service Office: 11830 Westline Industrial Drive, St. Louis, MO 63146. Periodicals postage paid at New York, NY, and additional mailing offices. Subscription prices are $274.00 per year (US individuals), $438.00 per year (US institutions), $300.00 per year (Canadian individuals), $535.00 per year (Canadian institutions), $383.00 per year (international individuals), $535.00 per year (international institutions), $138.00 per year (US students), and $189.00 per year (international students). International air speed delivery is included in all *Clinics* subscription prices. All prices are subject to change without notice. **POSTMASTER:** Send address changes to *Neurosurgery Clinics of North America*, Elsevier Periodicals Customer Service, 11830 Westline Industrial Drive, St. Louis, MO 63146. **Customer Service: 1-800-654-2452 (US and Canada). From outside the US and Canada, call 1-314-453-7041. Fax: 1-314-453-5170. E-mail: JournalsCustomerService-usa@elsevier.com (for print support)** and journalsonlinesupport-usa@elsevier.com (for online support).

Reprints. For copies of 100 or more, of articles in this publication, please contact the Commercial Reprints Department, Elsevier Inc., 360 Park Avenue South, New York, NY 10010-1710. Tel. (212) 633-3812; Fax: (212) 462-1935; email: reprints@elsevier.com.

Neurosurgery Clinics of North America is covered in *MEDLINE/PubMed (Index Medicus) EMBASE/Excerpta Medica, and Current Contents/Clinical Medicine (CC/CM)*.

Printed and bound by CPI Group (UK) Ltd, Croydon, CR0 4YY
Transferred to Digital Print 2011

Contributors

GUEST EDITORS

CHRISTOPHER J. WINFREE, MD
Department of Neurological Surgery,
Columbia University Medical Center,
New York, New York

ROBERT J. SPINNER, MD
Professor, Departments of Neurologic Surgery
and Orthopedics and Anatomy, Mayo Clinic,
Rochester, Minnesota

AUTHORS

BASSAM M.J. ADDAS, MBChB, FRCSC
Assistant Professor of Surgery, Division of
Neurosurgery, Department of Surgery, King
Abdulaziz University Hospital, Jeddah,
Kingdom of Saudi Arabia

GREGOR ANTONIADIS, MD, PhD
Professor of Neurosurgery, LOA, Department
of Neurosurgery, University of Ulm, Günzburg,
Germany

**ROLFE BIRCH, MChir, FRCS&P (Glas),
FRCS (Edin), FRCS (Eng)**
Royal National Orthopaedic Hospital,
Stanmore, United Kingdom

ALLEN T. BISHOP, MD
Professor and Consultant, Mayo Clinic,
Department of Orthopedic Surgery, Division
of Hand Surgery, Rochester, Minnesota

BRIAN T. CARLSEN, MD
Assistant Professor and Senior Associate
Consultant, Mayo Clinic, Division of Hand
Surgery, Rochester, Minnesota

THOMAS CARLSTEDT, PhD, MB
Visiting Professor, Imperial College, London;
and Professor, University College London,
United Kingdom; Foreign Adjunct Professor,
Karolinska Institutet, Stockholm, Sweden

GODARD C.W. DE RUITER, MD
Department of Neurosurgery, Leiden University
Medical Center, Leiden, The Netherlands

**JAMES M. ECKLUND, MD, FACS,
COL(Ret), MC**
Chairman, Department of Neurosciences,
Inova Fairfax Hospital, Falls Church, Virginia;
Professor of Surgery, Uniformed Services
University, Bethesda, Maryland; Professor of
Neurosurgery, George Washington University,
Washington, DC

CHRISTIAN W. HEINEN, MD
Department of Neurosurgery, University of
Ulm, Günzburg, Germany

DAVID G. KLINE, MD
Emeritus Chair and Boyd Professor of
Neurosurgery, Department of Neurosurgery,
Louisiana State University Health Sciences
Center; and Neurosurgery Clinic, Ochsner
Hospital, New Orleans, Louisiana

RALPH W. KÖNIG, MD, OA
Department of Neurosurgery, University of
Ulm, Günzburg, Germany

THOMAS KRETSCHMER, MD, PhD, OA
Department of Neurosurgery, University of
Ulm, Günzburg, Germany

GEOFFREY S.F. LING, MD, COL, MC
Professor and Vice Chairman, Neurology
Department, Uniformed Services University,
Bethesda, Maryland

MARTIJN J.A. MALESSY, MD, PhD
Department of Neurosurgery, Leiden University
Medical Center, Leiden, The Netherlands

RAJIV MIDHA, MD, MSc, FRSCS
Professor and Head of Neurosurgery, Division
of Neurosurgery, Department of Clinical
Neurosciences, Foothills Medical Center,
University of Calgary, Calgary, Alberta, Canada

WILLEM PONDAAG, MD
Department of Neurosurgery, Leiden University
Medical Center, Leiden, The Netherlands

HANS-PETER RICHTER, MD, PhD
Professor of Neurosurgery, Chairman,
Department of Neurosurgery, University of
Ulm, Günzburg, Germany

STEPHEN M. RUSSELL, MD
Assistant Professor of Neurosurgery,
Department of Neurosurgery, New York
University School of Medicine, New York,
New York

ALEXANDER Y. SHIN, MD
Professor and Consultant, Mayo Clinic,
Department of Orthopedic Surgery, Division of
Hand Surgery, Rochester, Minnesota

JAE W. SONG, MD
Department of Neurosurgery, New York
University School of Medicine, New York,
New York

ROBERT J. SPINNER, MD
Department of Neurologic Surgery; and
Department of Orthopedic Surgery, Mayo
Clinic, Rochester, Minnesota

R. MORGAN STUART, MD
Department of Neurological Surgery,
Columbia University Medical Center,
New York, New York

ANTHONY J. WINDEBANK, MD
Department of Neurology, Mayo Clinic,
Rochester, Minnesota

CHRISTOPHER J. WINFREE, MD, FACS
Assistant Professor of Neurological Surgery,
Columbia University Medical Center, New
York, New York

LYNDA J. YANG, MD, PhD
Assistant Professor of Surgery, Department
of Neurosurgery, University of Michigan School
of Medicine, Taubman Center, Ann Arbor,
Michigan

MICHAEL J. YASZEMSKI, MD, PhD
Department of Orthopedic Surgery, Mayo
Clinic, Rochester, Minnesota

Contents

Nerve transfers are becoming used increasingly for repair of severe nerve injures, especially brachial plexus injuries, where the proximal spinal nerve roots have been avulsed from the spinal cord. The procedure essentially involves the coaptation of a proximal foreign (donor) nerve to the distal denervated (recipient) nerve, so that the latter's end-organs will be reinnervated by the donated axons. Cortical plasticity appears to play an important physiologic role in the functional recovery of the reinnervated muscles. This article provides the indications for nerve transfer, principles for their use, and a comprehensive survey on various intraplexal and extraplexal nerves that have been used for transfer to repair clinical nerve injuries. Specific transfers to reanimate muscles denervated by the common patterns of brachial plexus are emphasized, including expected clinical outcomes based on the existing literature.

Traumatic avulsion of nerve roots from the spinal cord is a devastating event that usually occurs in the brachial plexus of young adults following motor vehicle or sports accidents or in newborn children during difficult childbirth. A strategy to restore motor function in the affected arm by reimplanting into the spinal cord the avulsed ventral roots or autologous nerve grafts connected distally to the avulsed roots has been developed. Surgical outcome is good and useful recovery in shoulder and proximal arm muscles occurs. Pain is alleviated with motor recovery but sensory improvement is poor when only motor conduits have been reconstructed. In experimental studies, restoration of sensory connections with general improvement in the outcome from this surgery is pursued.

Traumatic brachial plexus injuries are devastating and management is complex. Treatment involves a multidisciplinary approach. Primary reconstruction involves nerve repair, grafting, and transfer techniques. Secondary reconstruction includes microneurovascular free-functioning muscle transfer, tendon transfers, and arthrodesis to improve or restore function. These procedures are indicated when patients present more than 12 months from injury or when primary reconstruction procedures fail, and should focus on elbow flexion and shoulder stability. A free-functioning muscle transfer is often indicated for elbow flexion, with double free-functioning muscle transfers providing possible prehension. Shoulder reconstruction focuses on restoring stability to the glenohumeral joint and restoring abduction. This article outlines these techniques, their principles, and important details.

In the hands of the inexperienced, endoscopic carpal tunnel release bears a substantial risk for neurovascular injury. For those thoroughly trained in this technique, it is a fast and elegant but also more expensive way to achieve carpal tunnel release. If performed uneventfully, it minimizes trauma and avoids a substantial palmar skin incision. The authors think that some basic considerations are useful to prevent complications. This article focuses on some points that are relevant to the safe use of this technique.

Iatrogenic Nerve Injuries   73

Thomas Kretschmer, Christian W. Heinen, Gregor Antoniadis, Hans-Peter Richter, and Ralph W. König

As long as humans have been medically treated, unfortunate cases of inadvertent injury to nerves afflicted by the therapist have occurred. Most microsurgically treated iatrogenic nerve injuries occur directly during an operation. Certain nerves are at a higher risk than others, and certain procedures and regions of the body are more prone to sustaining nerve injury. A high degree of insecurity regarding the proper measures to take can be observed among medical practitioners. A major limiting factor in successful treatment is delayed referral for evaluation and reconstructive surgery. This article on iatrogenic nerve injuries intends to focus on relevant aspects of management from a nerve surgeon's perspective.

Nerve Tubes for Peripheral Nerve Repair   91

Godard C.W. de Ruiter, Robert J. Spinner, Michael J. Yaszemski, Anthony J. Windebank, and Martijn J.A. Malessy

The concept of the nerve tube has been a major topic of research in the field of peripheral nerve regeneration for more than 25 years. The first nerve tubes are currently available for clinical use. This article gives an overview of the experimental and clinical data on nerve tubes for peripheral nerve repair and critically analyzes the data on which the step from laboratory to clinical use is based. In addition, it briefly discusses the different modifications to the common single lumen nerve tubes that may improve the results of generation.

From the Battlefront: Peripheral Nerve Surgery in Modern Day Warfare   107

James M. Ecklund and Geoffrey S.F. Ling

Warfare historically causes a large number of peripheral nerve injuries. During the current global war on terror, an increased use of advanced regional anesthesia techniques appears to have significantly reduced pain syndromes that have been previously reported with missile-induced nerve injuries. Additionally, a new program has been established to develop advanced prosthetic devises that can interface with neural tissue to obtain direct neural control. As this technology matures, the functional restoration gained from these new generation prosthetic devices may exceed that which can be obtained by standard nerve repair techniques.

Peripheral Nerve Pain

Neurostimulation Techniques for Painful Peripheral Nerve Disorders   111

R. Morgan Stuart and Christopher J. Winfree

Disorders of the peripheral nervous system often present a unique challenge to the clinician or surgeon, because the neuropathic pain associated with them can be extremely resistant to typical pain treatments. Painful peripheral nerve disorders often have pain in a particular peripheral nerve distribution, and thus an optimal treatment modality is one that delivers targeted relief to the precise distribution of the pain. To that end, peripheral nerve stimulation (PNS) has undergone several refinements in recent years. New types of stimulation, such as techniques for cranial nerve stimulation and spinal nerve root stimulation (SNRS), have enabled the treatment of painful peripheral nerve problems that until fairly recently were either untreatable or poorly treated with traditional spinal cord stimulation (SCS) techniques. In this article, PNS techniques are described in detail for the stimulation of the occipital and trigeminal nerves for intractable craniofacial pain, as well as emerging techniques for the selective stimulation of spinal nerve roots and subcutaneous peripheral nerve stimulation. The increasing spectrum of disorders and pain syndromes amenable to PNS also is discussed.

Translational Peripheral Nerve Research

Peripheral nerve regeneration research has unfolded a wealth of basic science knowledge in the last century. Today, that knowledge has become the fundamental groundwork for evolving clinical applications to treat peripheral nerve defects. This article discusses two clinical applications that have been investigated thoroughly in the laboratory setting for decades and recently tested in the clinical setting: nerve allotransplantation to graft nerve defects, and brief electrical stimulation to promote nerve regeneration. It also discusses the generation of Thy-1-XFP transgenic mice, which express fluorescent proteins in the nervous system and provide new avenues for investigating peripheral nerve regeneration.

Neurosurgery Clinics of North America

THE CLINICS ARE NOW AVAILABLE ONLINE!

Access your subscription at:
www.theclinics.com

Preface

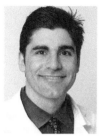 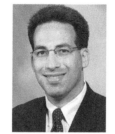

Christopher J. Winfree, MD   Robert J. Spinner, MD
Guest Editors

Consecutive issues of *Neurosurgery Clinics of North America* highlight "what's new" in peripheral nerve surgery. Significant recent advances have been made in the management of peripheral nerve entrapments and tumors (featured in Part I), as well as injuries (including wartime injuries) and neuropathic pain (featured in Part II). Novel experimental strategies, which hold tremendous promise for translational applications (reviewed in Part II), are currently being tested.

We fully acknowledge that "what's new" is not necessarily "what's better." Time, along with well-designed outcome studies, will determine this. Certain things that are new turn out to be fads or even failures. Sometimes, what's new is realizing that the old paradigm is better. Over time, some new developments automatically and appropriately become adopted as major advances. We also realize that people react differently to new ideas—some with infectious enthusiasm, some with cautious optimism, and others with frank skepticism. Therefore, we have tried to feature specific controversial topics

in a balanced fashion, allowing the reader to be the judge.

We present this two-part series with excitement. It represents a celebration of peripheral nerve surgery—its rich past and its bright future.

Christopher J. Winfree, MD
Department of Neurological Surgery
Columbia University Medical Center
710 West 168th Street
New York, NY 10032, USA

Robert J. Spinner, MD
Departments of Neurologic Surgery
and Orthopedics
Mayo Clinic
200 First Street West
Rochester, MN 55905, USA

E-mail addresses:
cjw12@columbia.edu (C.J. Winfree)
spinner.robert@mayo.edu (R.J. Spinner)

doi:10.1016/j.nec.2008.09.002

neurosurgery.theclinics.com

Obstetric Brachial Plexus Injuries

Martijn J.A. Malessy, MD, PhD*, Willem Pondaag, MD

KEYWORDS
- Brachial plexus • Obstetric brachial plexus lesion
- Brachial plexus repair • Nerve surgery

An obstetric brachial plexus lesion (OBPL) is thought to be caused by traction to the brachial plexus during labour.[1,2] In most cases, delivery of the upper shoulder is blocked by the mother's symphysis (shoulder dystocia). If additional traction is applied to the child's head, the angle between neck and shoulder may be forcefully widened, further stretching the ipsilateral brachial plexus.

The incidence of OBPL varies from 0.42 to 2.9 per 1000 births in prospective studies.[3–5] Risk factors that have been identified for the occurrence of OBPL reflect the disproportion between the child and the birth canal. The main fetal risk factor is macrosomia;[6,7] maternal factors include gestational diabetes and multiparity.[6] Shoulder dystocia and assisted delivery by forceps or vacuum cup are well-known risk factors for the development of OBPL.[6] A less common delivery pattern concerns infants, usually with low birth weight, born in a breech position. This pattern carries a high risk for root avulsion.[8]

The debate is ongoing about whether OBPL is preventable and whether the obstetrician can be held responsible. This debate is fed by numerous malpractice suits in which large sums of money are compensated.[9] Case reports of spontaneous deliveries without traction applied to the child during labor with the occurrence of brachial plexus injury have been reported, suggesting that these injuries may occur in the absence of negligently performed delivery maneuvers.[10] The upper brachial plexus is most commonly affected, resulting in paresis of the supraspinatus, infraspinatus, deltoid, and biceps muscles, as first described by Erb and Duchenne. Typically, in the C5-C6 lesion type, the affected arm is resting on the surface in adduction, internal rotation, and extension. The wrist and fingers are continuously flexed when C7 is also damaged (**Fig. 1**). Hand function is additionally impaired in approximately 15 % of patients;[3,11,12] isolated injury to the lower plexus (Déjèrine-Klumpke type) is rare.[13]

The traction injury may vary from neurapraxia to axonotmesis, to neurotmesis, or to avulsion of rootlets from the spinal cord.[14] The severity of neural damage can only be assessed by evaluation of recovery in the course of time, because nerve lesions of different severity initially present with the same clinical features. Neurapraxia and axonotmesis eventually result in complete or near-complete recovery. Neurotmesis and root avulsion, on the other hand, result in permanent loss of arm function and, in time, development of skeletal malformations, cosmetic deformities, behavioral problems, and socioeconomic limitations.[15–19]

NATURAL HISTORY

The prognosis of OPBL is generally considered to be good, with complete or almost-complete spontaneous recovery in more than 90% of patients.[20–25] However, these data are based on a limited number of series,[26,27] without considering important methodologic aspects of these studies. In a systematic literature review, we discussed the methodologic flaws in the available natural history studies.[28] We found that no study presented a prospective, population-based cohort that was scored with a proper scoring system with adequate follow-up. In other words, no scientifically sound evidence exists to support the common perception of complete spontaneous recovery

Department of Neurosurgery, Leiden University Medical Center, P.O. Box 9600, 2300 RC Leiden, The Netherlands
* Corresponding author.
E-mail address: malessy@lumc.nl (M.J.A. Malessy).

Neurosurg Clin N Am 20 (2009) 1–14
doi:10.1016/j.nec.2008.07.024
1042-3680/08/$ – see front matter © 2008 Elsevier Inc. All rights reserved.

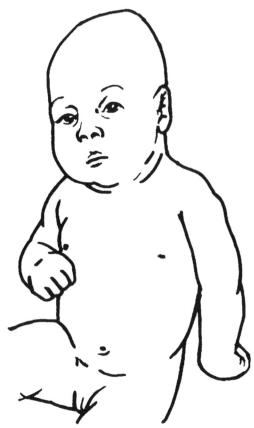

Fig. 1. An infant who has a C5-C6-C7 lesion. The affected left arm is held in adduction, internal rotation, and extension. The wrist and fingers are continuously flexed.

from OBPL. The often-cited excellent prognosis may be too optimistic. Analysis of the most methodologically sound studies led us to estimate the percentage of children who have residual deficits to be 20% to 30%.

NEUROPATHOPHYSIOLOGY

In OBPL infants, the damaged nerves are usually not completely ruptured, in the sense that a gap exists between two stumps (neurotmesis), which is most likely caused by the gradual exertion of traction forces over a small distance that act during a long period. The two crucial factors that determine good functional recovery are the number of damaged axons that successfully elongate past the lesion site and their routing. Axonal outgrowth and restoration of connections with their original motor or sensory end organs can only take place when the basal lamina tubes surrounding the axons, which are in this context the crucial anatomic structures, remain intact. The distance from the lesion site, which in OBPL is almost always at root and trunk level, to the end organ determines the length of the time required for recovery. Proximal muscles recover, therefore, at an earlier stage than more distally located ones. Recovery of predominantly axonometic OBP lesions is usually seen within the first 3 to 4 months of life.

When the traction lesion is severe, the basal lamina tubes are ruptured, but the perineurium and epineurium remain more or less intact. Outgrowing axons may not then end up directly in any tube. Typical for the OBPL is that the stretched and damaged nerve forms a "neuroma-in-continuity" (ie, a tangled mass of connective scar tissue and outgrowing, branching axons). The local environment encountered by the axonal growth cone may impede outgrowth and may ultimately block the restoration of axonal continuity. Even in the most severe OBPL C5-C6 lesions, at least some axons will pass through the neuroma-in-continuity and reach the tubes distal to the lesion site. The number of axons, though, may not be sufficient to yield a clinically significant functional result. The number of axons that will not pass the lesion site depends on the severity of the lesion, which is determined by the magnitude and angle of the exerted traction forces. A minimum number of axons should reconnect with an end organ to regain function. In addition, adequate recovery requires a minimum of axons that should be properly routed to their original end organ. We presume that those axons in the OBPL neuroma-in-continuity are particularly prone to abnormal branching and misrouting. Because the direction of outgrowth after severe lesions is essentially random,[29] outgrowing axons growing through a neuroma-in-continuity are likely to end up in the wrong tube. Each OBPL case is unique on an axonal level in that the number of ruptured axons and basal laminal tubes differ for each intraplexal element, which subsequently leads to the wide variety in level of functional recovery found in individual cases. Branching and misrouting can also explain cocontraction,[30] a typical feature of OBPL at a later age, in which shoulder abduction and elbow flexion, or elbow flexion and extension, become irreversibly linked.

The most severe lesion type, which is specifically related to traction to the spinal nerves forming the brachial plexus, is a root avulsion. The result is a complete discontinuity of the neural connections of the central nervous system to the peripheral nervous system. Outgrowth of axons, and thus neuroma formation or misrouting, will not take place in the case of a root avulsion.

In addition to the inadequate number of outgrowing axons and misrouting that may reduce functional regeneration, improper central motor programming may occur.[31] The formation of motor programs may fail in OBPL for various reasons. First, OBPL causes deafferentation and weakness; many functions in the central nervous system depend on afferent input in a specific time window or else they are not formed correctly. Second, aberrant outgrowth of motor axons may present the central nervous system with conflicting information. A motor command for shoulder abduction may, for instance, cause elbow flexion in addition to abduction, through misrouted motor axons. The resulting feedback may well hamper the formation of a selective abduction program, because the central nervous system probably has no way to identify the "misbehaving" motor units.[32,33] Third, sensory axons might also be prone to misrouting, compounding the problem. A final hurdle for the central nervous system may be the severity of paresis. In such cases, the only way to effect certain movements may be through "trick movements" (such as scapular rotation instead of glenohumeral rotation), which then represent a functional adaptation.

CONSERVATIVE TREATMENT THE FIRST FEW MONTHS OF LIFE

In the past, the tendency has been to immobilize the arm directly after birth to prevent secondary damage to the injured nerve elements of the brachial plexus. It is highly unlikely that secondary damage to the brachial plexus can occur during the passive movements of the arm in a physiologic range of motion during exercises or care taking. We advocate the early and frequent mobilization of the affected extremity to prevent joint contracture and enhance the potential for future recovery. Not only does no scientific proof exist that immobilization is of any benefit to the nerve regeneration process but joint contracture formation might be detrimental to the final functional outcome when contractures limit the effective contraction of reinnervated muscles. It may also lead to improper modeling of the joints, of which the glenohumeral joint is most frequently affected.[18] Contracture formation may start as early as 2 to 3 weeks after birth. These typically restrict internal rotation, flexion, and pronation of the upper limb. Exercises that focus on prevention of contracture formation and optimization of joint mobility consist of passive external rotation in adduction and supination with an elbow flexed at 90°, just to the point where a certain tension can be felt. The arm should be held in this position for a few seconds and then released. This passive movement should be repeated frequently during one session. We advise the parents to mobilize the affected arm as frequently as possible during the day, but at least every time the diaper is changed. In addition, we recommend that the parents move both arms in a symmetric fashion. In this way, the parents can use the unaffected arm range of motion as a reference value and therapy target of reach for the affected arm. The joint mobility should be evaluated every week by a specialized child physiotherapist.

SURGICAL TREATMENT
Indications

Surgery should be restricted to severe cases in which spontaneous restoration of function is not likely to occur (ie, in neurotmesis or root avulsions).[14] The clinical difficulty lies in the ability to distinguish these patients from those who have similar deficits but who have a high likelihood of spontaneous recovery. At present, the earliest accepted indication of the severity of the lesion can be obtained at 3 months of age. Paralysis of the biceps muscle at 3 months is associated with a poor prognosis[34] and is considered an indication for nerve surgery by some investgators.[35–39] However, biceps paralysis at age 3 months does not preclude satisfactory spontaneous recovery.[40–43] Additionally, biceps muscle testing may not be reliable in infants.[43–45] Alternative tests[39,44,46] are complex or are done at an even later age. These difficulties in the diagnostic process may also lead to parental distress.[47] We are in favor of concentrating the treatment of severe OBPL in specialized referral centers. Early diagnosis of severe OBPL lesions and admission to a specialized center opens opportunities to start appropriate and rigorous child physiotherapy or (appropriately) early surgery, if necessary.

Electromyography and Prognosis

Ancillary testing, in particular, electromyography (EMG), is not considered reliable enough for prognostication of OBPL.[32,48] A needle EMG might seem a useful tool in this respect, but at present, its role is debated. A main reason for this is that EMG findings may be discordant with clinical findings at 3 months of age, at which the biceps test is performed.[37] In a paralytic biceps brachii muscle, the expected findings are an absence of motor unit potentials (MUPs) and the presence of positive sharp waves or fibrillation potentials (to be called "denervational changes"). But in a typical OBPL case, MUPs are present and denervation is absent in a paralytic biceps muscle at 3 months of age. This confusing finding has been noted by others,[49,50] and may have contributed to the opinion that the EMG is not useful in OBPL.[24,51] We previously outlined several possible explanations for "inactive MUPs," (ie, MUPs in a paralytic muscle),[32] which suggest that the presence of inactive MUPs may depend on time after injury because they reflect incomplete outgrowth of damaged axons and the formation of motor programs in the central nervous system.

Spontaneous recovery of useful extremity function has been observed in patients who do not have elbow flexion at 3 months of age.[43] In one study, even 20 of 28 infants who had no biceps function at 3 months had developed biceps contraction at 6 months.[41] Together with our findings[52] that MUPs can almost always be found in the biceps muscle at 3 months, this finding strongly suggests that the age of 3 months does not represent a stable state in OBPL. In fact, the outgrowing axons may well have only just arrived in the various muscles, and the central nervous system may not yet have learned to cope with the situation. In nerve lesions in adults, one may expect all motor programs to be ready and waiting for the restoration of peripheral connections. In OBPL, axonal outgrowth may only be the starting point for restoration of function because formation of central nervous system motor programs may only commence after enough axons have arrived at their muscle targets. At the same time, forming such central motor programs may be more difficult and thus may take longer than in healthy children because the central nervous system must somehow take aberrant outgrowth and the confusing feedback it causes into account. Faced with a degree of inescapable co-contraction, it may not be easy to program effective elbow flexion, abduction, or rotation. In this hypothetic view, the age of 3 months may well be the worst period imaginable to correlate the EMG with clinical findings: it is late enough to show evidence of axonal outgrowth, but too early for the brain to control contraction efficiently. Therefore, the role of the EMG for prognosis at 3 months remains undetermined at present. We showed that severe cases of OBPL can be identified reliably at 1 month of age based on clinical findings and needle EMG of the biceps.[52] These findings will be reported in full after independent validation, which is currently in progress.

For less extreme cases (ie, most OBPL cases), the challenge lies in predicting whether function will be better after spontaneous outgrowth through a neuroma-in-continuity, resulting in reinnervation through tangled paths, or after nerve grafting, in which the grafts serve as a straight path that can be targeted. Results achieved by surgery are claimed to be superior to the outcome in conservatively treated patients who have equally severe lesions.[37,42,53] However, this comparison relies on historical controls;[54] no randomized study has been performed.[55,56] The best way to answer this question may be by way of a controlled trial comparing nerve surgery to spontaneous recovery. In view of the current standard of treatment practice, it seems extremely difficult to perform such a prospective randomized trial.

Selection for Surgery

In the Leiden University Medical Center, surgery for OBPL is rarely performed before 3 months of age (for anaesthesiologic reasons) but almost always before the age of 7 months. In selecting infants for surgery, we seek to identify all cases of neurotmesis or avulsion. Infants are selected for surgery when external shoulder rotation and elbow flexion with supination remain paralytic after a 3- to 4-month period to await spontaneous recovery. Impaired hand function is an absolute indication for nerve surgery as soon as the infant turns 3 months old.[57] If the quality of shoulder and elbow joint movements is doubtful, surgical exploration is performed hoping that errors would consist of not finding neurotmesis or avulsion during surgery rather than letting such lesions go unoperated. Preoperative ancillary investigations in all patients consist of ultrasound of diaphragm excursions to assess phrenic nerve function and CT myelography under general anesthesia to detect root avulsions (**Fig. 2**).[58,59]

Surgical Exposure

In OBPLs, supraclavicular brachial plexus exploration is the first step, to localize the site and extent of the lesion. In most cases, this exposure will suffice for proper evaluation and reconstruction, if needed. The supraclavicular incision runs parallel and superior to the clavicle at the basis of the lateral cervical triangle. After opening the deep fascia colli media, the phrenic nerve is identified in its course over the ventral surface of the anterior scalene muscle. The site where the phrenic nerve crosses the lateral border of the anterior scalene muscle consistently lies on top of the spinal nerve C5 where it emerges from the C4-C5 foramen; hence, it is a reliable surgical landmark. The phrenic nerve is then neurolysed in its trajectory running on top of the anterior scalene muscle to allow a medial transposition without traction on the phrenic nerve. Resection or partial resection of the scalene muscles is indicated in order to make a good inspection of the proximal, intraforaminal, part of the spinal nerves possible. Because such proximal exposure involves a risk for opening

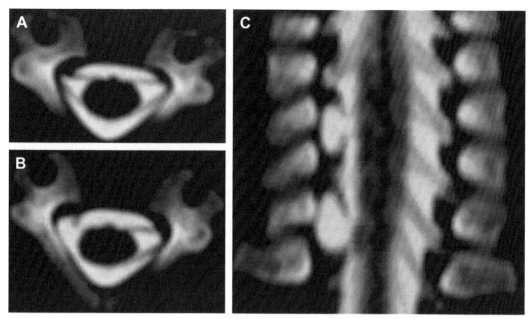

Fig. 2. CT myelography. (*A*) Normal CT myelography. (*B*) Avulsed root on the right side. Note the absence of root filaments and the small pseudomeningocele. (*C*) Coronal reconstruction of the CT myelogram demonstrating right-sided pseudomeningoceles.

a pseudomeningocele that extends extraforaminally, care should be taken to identify such pseudomeningocele on CT myelography or MRI. The omohyoid muscle is identified as the caudal aspect of the exploration. We do not resect the omohyoid muscle but instead, mobilize it and retract it downward to the clavicle. Occasionally, the transverse cervical vein and artery are ligated and divided. The suprascapular nerve (SSN) originating at the lateral side of the superior trunk normally follows a slightly oblique cranial-caudal course to the scapular notch. Caudal displacement of the superior trunk changes this course in a more or less horizontal direction.

Occasionally, the lesion extends to the infraclavicular part of the brachial plexus. The infraclavicular brachial plexus may be surgically exposed in several ways. The major and minor pectoral muscles cover the brachial plexus, which runs medial to the coracobrachial muscle and short head of biceps brachii muscle. A straight incision is made above the deltoid-pectoral groove. The major pectoral muscle is retracted downwards to expose the infraclavicular brachial plexus. The minor pectoral muscle is alternately retracted upward and downward allowing inspection of the entire infraclavicular plexus. The brachial plexus, with accompanying vessels, is initially identified at the inferior border of the pectoralis minor muscle. To facilitate retroclavicular exposure, if indicated, the retroclavicular space can be widened for inspection by upward clavicular retraction by an assistant or a suspended, table-mounted retractor. An alternating supra- and infraclavicular view allows dissection or repair of the retroclavicular nerve bundles (**Fig. 3**).

In its upper infraclavicular course, the posterior cord runs lateral and posterior, rather than medial and posterior, to the lateral cord. The latter course is frequently depicted incorrectly in schematic anatomic drawings. The axillary nerve runs through the quadrilateral space above the latissimus dorsi and teres major tendons. This nerve can be identified more easily by external rotation of the humerus.

When nerve transfers are applied, the donor nerves are dissected free. An absolute imperative of donor nerves is that these nerves have normal function. Their identification and function can be tested with direct electric stimulation. The accessory nerve (XIN) can be identified on the medial-anterior surface of the trapezius muscle. The nerve gives off a branch to the superior part of the trapezius muscle, which has to be kept intact. The accessory nerve is dissected free distally as far in its course as possible and cut. The proximal stump is then passed through the fascia colli media. In this way, a direct coaptation with the SSN can almost always be performed. The medial pectoral nerves can be identified running below the minor and major pectoral muscles. Because the medial pectoral nerve originates from the

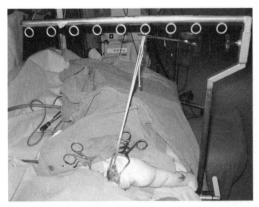

Fig. 3. Exposure of the retroclavicular part of the brachial plexus can be easily improved by pulling the clavicle upwards by a lace that is attached to a bar above the operating table. An additional incision is not needed. When using these additional, table-mounted retractor systems, care must be taken to guard against positioning injuries, with the use of sufficient padding between the system and the patient.

medial cord,[60] its function is intact in C5-C6 or C5-C6-C7 lesions. Nerve stimulation is an indispensable step in the identification of the medial pectoral nerve because small vessels may occasionally have an almost similar aspect and course. Routinely, two individual medial pectoral nerve branches exist. They should be cut as distally as possible and then transferred laterally to the musculocutaneous nerve (MCN). Depending on the cross-sectional area of the medial pectoral nerve branches, the MCN is cut completely or only partially. Direct pectoral-musculocutaneous coaptation is feasible in most cases.

We previously described the technique for intercostal nerve (ICN) transfer in adults.[61] We apply the same surgical technique in OBPL infants. In short, three ICNs are dissected through an undulating skin incision from the inferior border of the major pectoral muscle to the costosternal junction. The ICNs are transected as close as possible to the sternum to obtain sufficient length to be tunneled to the axilla for direct coaptation to the MCN.

Surgical Assessment of the Severity of the Lesion

Surgery is performed under general anesthesia without muscle blocking agents. The brachial plexus is exposed in the lateral neck triangle through a straight incision parallel to the clavicle. Depending on the extent of injury, the infraclavicular part is also exposed. The severity of the lesion of each clinically involved spinal nerve is subsequently assessed. A distinction is made between axonotmesis, neurotmesis, and root avulsion based on (1) inspection of the status of nerve continuity at the intraforaminal level in combination with the presence or absence of root filaments on CT myelography; (2) the extent and location of neuroma formation; (3) selective electric stimulation of all the involved spinal nerves using a bipolar forceps in combination with a 2.5-Hz pulse generator with increasing voltage (maximum 6 V).

A spinal nerve root is considered avulsed when the nerve at the intraforaminal and juxtaforaminal levels exhibits root filaments, the dorsal root ganglion is visible, neuroma formation is absent, and no muscle contractions occur following direct stimulation. In most spinal nerves, these findings correspond with the absence of root filaments as demonstrated by CT myelography. Avulsed roots are cut as proximally as possible. When the dorsal root ganglion can be morphologically identified, it is dissected from the ventral root and removed. Following confirmation by frozen section of the presence of ganglion cells, one may be certain that the distal stump consisted only of the ventral root. This ventral root can be the target for nerve grafting, or the ventral root can be attached to a qualitatively good nerve stump directly, without a nerve graft.

A spinal nerve is considered neurotmetic when the following features are present: a normal appearance at the intraforaminal level, a clear increase of the cross-sectional diameter at the juxtaforaminal level, abundant epineural fibrosis, loss of fascicular continuity, increased consistency, and increase in the length of the nerve elements with concomitant distal displacement of the trunk divisions. Electric stimulation of the spinal nerve proximal to the neuroma might cause weak muscle contractions that are detectable with palpation but are not strong enough to move the limb. Resection of neurotmetic tissue is performed, and the proximal and distal stumps are prepared for nerve reconstruction.

A spinal nerve is considered axonometic when neurolysis reveals no substantial increase in the cross-sectional diameter, only limited epineural fibrosis and intact fascicular continuity. Furthermore, on C5 stimulation, abduction with movement of the limb and some external rotation should be present, and on C6 stimulation, elbow flexion against gravity with supination should be found. These movements, of course, will only occur if sufficient time has elapsed for spontaneous recovery to occur, which is often not the case with fairly early surgery at 3 to 5 months. Axonotmetic nerves are left in situ because spontaneous nerve regeneration is in process, although as yet clinically not clearly apparent. Axonotmesis is confirmed by the occurrence of good spontaneous recovery after at least 2 years of follow-up.

Intraoperative Electrodiagnostic Studies

In adults, recording of intraoperative nerve action potentials (NAP) and evoked compound motor action potentials (CMAP) is advocated to distinguish objectively between nonconducting and recovering lesions.[62,63] The presence of a NAP across the lesion site requires at least 3000 to 4000 nerve fibers with a diameter more than 5 μm. The presence of these fibers in a recovering nerve indicates that spontaneous functional recovery will take place, and that, therefore, resection and grafting are not indicated.[64]

We analyzed the results of intraoperative NAP and CMAP recordings in 95 patients who had OBPL to assess the predictive values for the diagnosis of axonotmesis, neurotmesis, avulsion, or normal spinal nerves, respectively.[65] We found statistically significant differences among diagnosis groups. For the individual patient, however, a clinically useful cutoff point for NAP and CMAP recordings to differentiate between avulsion, neurotmesis, axonotmesis, and normal could not be found. The sensitivity for an absent NAP or CMAP was too low for clinical use. Intraoperative NAP and CMAP recordings, therefore, do not add to the decision making during surgery. Direct electric stimulation remains important to obtain a nonquantitative evaluation of the presence of axons in a regenerating nerve segment.

Surgical Reconstruction

The first goal of nerve repair is restoration of hand function if necessary; the second priority is restoration of elbow flexion, and the third goal is recovery of shoulder movements.[57] The sources of outgrowing axons for reinnervation are viable proximal nerve stumps, which we evaluate with frozen section examination. The total quantity of myelin in the entire cross-sectional area of the donor stump, which corresponds to the viability of the proximal stump, is expressed semiquantitatively: (1) less than 25%; (2) 25% to 50%; (3) 50% to 75%; (4) more than 75%.[66] The neuropathologist can additionally assess the presence of ganglion cells (indicative of total avulsion) and fibrosis/neuroma in the proximal and distal stumps. In our center, proximal stumps are only used as an outlet for nerve grafting and thus, are considered viable when the total myelin quantity is greater than or equal to 50%.

In most cases, nerve grafts are led out from a viable proximal nerve stump to distal target stumps after resection of a neuroma-in-continuity (**Fig. 4**). The preferred option in the case of a root avulsion is direct coaptation (so without the use a graft) between an available proximal nerve stump and the avulsed root (intraplexal nerve transfer) (**Fig. 5**). In such cases, the ventral and dorsal roots are separated, and the dorsal root ganglion is resected before direct coaptation or nerve grafting. When the number of proximal stumps is limited, intraplexal transfer or nerve grafting is used to reinnervate the hand and extra-intraplexal nerve transfers are performed to restore shoulder function and elbow flexion. A direct coaptation without a nerve graft is performed in cases in which the ICNs, medial pectoral, or spinal accessory nerves are used as the donor nerves.

Selection of the distal target stumps is determined by the aforementioned goals. For that reason, the first goal of hand function restoration is pursued by neurotization of C8, T1, inferior trunk, or middle trunk, aiming at restoration of median or ulnar nerve–innervated functions. Preferably, a direct coaptation to C8 without a nerve graft is performed (**Fig. 6**).[57]

The second priority is restoration of elbow flexion; the anterior division of the superior trunk, the lateral cord, or the MCN is chosen as the target nerve. The third goal is to recover shoulder movements and involved neurotization of the posterior division of the superior trunk, the suprascapular, or the axillary nerve. If possible, a graft is led out from C5 to the SSN to reanimate external rotation. The XIN–SSN transfer is performed when the available stumps have been used for nerve reconstruction, aiming at reanimation of the hand or biceps muscle. In all patients, both sural nerves are harvested as grafts, a procedure that is routinely performed with the aid of an endoscope (**Fig. 7**). In addition, the cutaneous cervical plexus or the cutaneous nerves of the arm or forearm are used in some cases.

Postoperative Treatment

Postoperatively, the child's upper body is placed in a prefabricated bay cast for a period of 2 weeks to limit movements of the head and affected arm. Patients are examined at our outpatient clinic at 6-month intervals. The active and passive range of joint movements is noted in degrees and Medical Research Council (MRC) grade. In addition, the Mallet score[67] is assessed to evaluate shoulder function and the Raimondi hand score is assessed to evaluate hand function.[68]

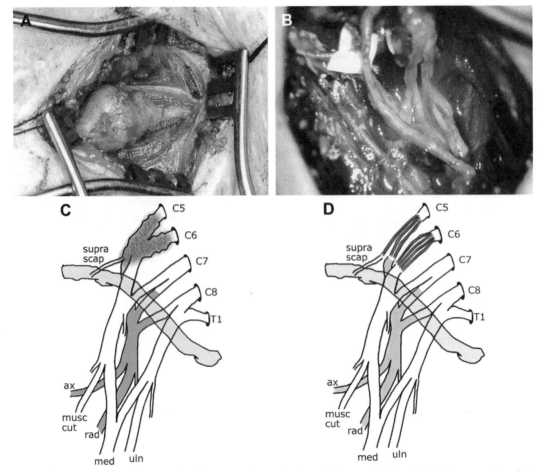

Fig. 4. (*A*) Intraoperative photograph of neuroma-in-continuity of the superior trunk. (*B*) Intraoperative photograph of nerve grafting of the spinal nerve C5 to the posterior division superior trunk and SSN and C6 to the anterior division superior trunk. (*C*) The most common lesion type: supraclavicular neuroma-in-continuity of the superior trunk. (*D*) Nerve grafting after resection of the neuroma of the spinal nerve C5 to the posterior division superior trunk and SSN and C6 to the anterior division superior trunk. ax, axillary nerve; med, median nerve; musc, musculocutaneous nerve; rad, radial nerve; supra scap, suprascapular nerve; uln, ulnar nerve.

RESULTS OF NERVE SURGERY
Shoulder Function

The results of nerve repairs to improve shoulder function have been published in several series, from which at first glance it can be concluded that global shoulder function recovery is good.[35,38,42,69,70] We performed a study (n = 86) that focused on the recovery of true glenohumeral external rotation as a solitary movement in to determine specific factors affecting recovery after neurotization of the SSN (**Table 1**).[71] During the neurologic evaluation of these children, trick movements were eliminated for a clean comparison of two surgical techniques and of other prognostic factors (**Fig. 8**). We found that only 20% of the patients gained more than a 20° range of true external rotation and that restoration of true

glenohumeral external rotation failed in as many as 41% of the patients. In contrast to this disappointing result of true external rotation, functional evaluation showed that 87% of the patients could reach their mouths and 75% of children could reach the backs of their heads, which illustrates the great ability of the infants to compensate for their limited true external rotation by thoracoscapular movements. We found no difference between nerve grafting C5-SSN and nerve transfer of XIN to SSN.

Elbow Flexion

In the previously mentioned cohort, biceps muscle force against gravity or more was gained in 92% of patients.[71] In most of these patients, nerve grafting had been performed. Recently, we analyzed

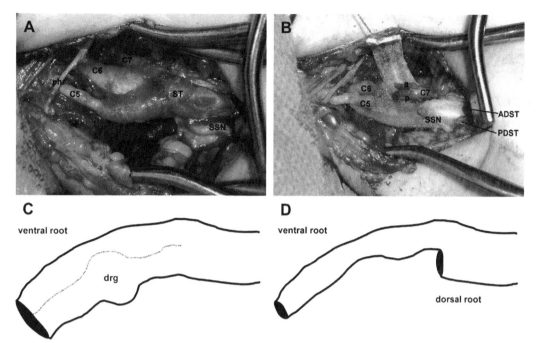

Fig. 5. (A) Intraoperative photo showing neuroma of the upper trunk. phr, phrenic nerve; ST, superior trunk. (B) After resection of the upper trunk, the ventral and dorsal rootlets of C7 are separated. a, anterior root filaments C7; p, posterior root filaments C7; ADST, anterior division superior trunk; PDST, posterior division superior trunk. (C) The structure of the avulsed root. drg, dorsal root ganglion. (D) After separation of ventral and dorsal roots, the dorsal root ganglion is resected.

30 consecutive patients (1995–2005) in whom nerve transfers for biceps reanimation had been applied (data not yet published). From 1995 to 2000, only intercostal-musculocutaneous nerve (ICN-MCN) transfers were performed, and from 2001 to 2005, the pectoral-musculocutaneous nerve (PEC-MCN) transfer was preferentially applied, when the C8/T1 trajectory to the inferior trunk was intact. In 15 of 16 ICN-MCN transfers, three ICNs were coapted directly to the MCN; in one patient, a 1-cm graft proved necessary. In all patients with PEC-MCN transfers, we were able to perform a direct coaptation. Elbow flexion greater than or equal to MRC 3 was achieved in 87% of patients after a mean follow-up of 40 months. The results in the PEC-MCN group were better than those of the ICN-MCN group (93% versus 81%, respectively), which may be explained by the more severe brachial plexus lesions that were included in the ICN-MCN group (8/16 patients in the ICN-MCN group had a flail arm). In the ICN-MCN group, one secondary surgery was performed (a Steindler flexorplasty). No adverse effects were noted in either group. We did not see any rib cage deformity after ICN-MCN transfer. Such deformities have been occasionally mentioned by some colleagues, but we are not aware of any reports in the literature. We think that the crucial factor for avoiding rib cage deformity is to leave the periosteum of the ribs untouched during dissection of the ICNs. In this way, the growth of the ribs of the infant remains undisturbed over time.

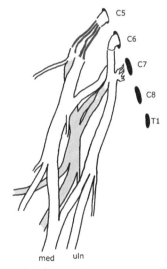

Fig. 6. Example of reconstruction of hand function: grafting C5-superior trunk and direct coaptation C6-C8. med, median nerve; uln, ulnar nerve.

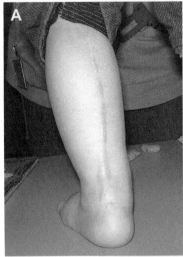
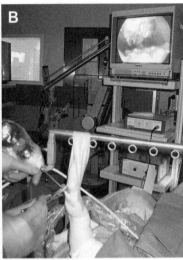
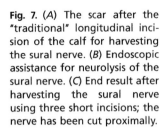
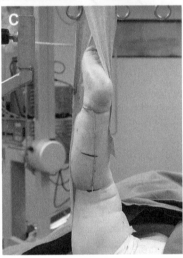

Fig. 7. (*A*) The scar after the "traditional" longitudinal incision of the calf for harvesting the sural nerve. (*B*) Endoscopic assistance for neurolysis of the sural nerve. (*C*) End result after harvesting the sural nerve using three short incisions; the nerve has been cut proximally.

These results correspond well to the few reports in literature. Kawabata[72] reported the results of 31 ICN-MCN transfers in OBPL patients: 94% reached greater than or equal to MRC 3. For the PEC-MCN transfer, a success rate of 88% greater than or equal to MRC3 was reported by Blaauw.[73] The transfer of a single fascicle of the ulnar nerve to the biceps motor branch has been proposed by some investigators as alternative intraplexal transfer, after satisfactory results in adults with this technique were published.[74,75] We have included this technique in our overall surgical strategy but feel that indications in OBPL infants may be limited, especially because the ICN-MCN and PEC-MCN transfers are almost always an option and provide satisfying results.

Recovery of Hand Function

The objective of surgical treatment of the infant who has a flail arm is significantly different from that in adult brachial plexus lesions. The main target is to establish the ability to use the affected hand to assist in bimanual activity. Combined with good elbow flexion, strong finger flexion is mandatory for a supportive role in the bimanual execution of daily life tasks. Without reanimation of the hand, the maximal function that can be obtained is the use of the affected limb as a "hook." In the past, reanimation of hand function in adults who had a total brachial plexus lesion has been tried, but it did not result in useful function.[76] Because of better nerve regeneration and neural plasticity in infants compared with adult patients, restoration of hand function in OBPL infants is feasible. The primary aim of surgery in patients who have a flail arm due to OBPL is, therefore, restoration of hand function. In our OBPL series, we identified and subsequently analyzed 16 patients who had a flail arm, in whom discontinuity of the outflow of the spinal nerves C7, C8, and T1 was

Table 1
Retrospective analysis of results at the Leiden University Medical Center

Subject	n	Year	Inclusion Criteria	Results
External rotation	86	1-1-1990 to 12-31-2000	Surgical reconstruction of SSN function Grafting C5-SSN or transfer XIN-SSN Follow-up: 3 years	20% true external rotation >20° 87% can reach mouth 75% can reach back of head 94% elbow flexion ≥ MRC 3
Elbow flexion	20	1-1-1995 to 12-31-2005	Nerve transfer for elbow flexion ICN-MCN or PEC-MCN transfer Follow-up: 2 years	86% elbow flexion ≥ MRC 3 PEC-MCN: 93% ICN-MCN: 81%
Hand function	16	1-1-1990 to 07-01-2002	Reconstruction of C8 and T1 Follow-up: 3 years (n = 15), 2 years (n = 1)	69% Raimondi hand score ≥ 3

Abbreviations: ICN-MCN, intercostal-musculocutaneous nerve; PEC-MCN, pectoral-musculocutaneous nerve.

present due to avulsion injury or neurotmetic parts of the outflow were resected, followed by neurotization of C8/T1/inferior trunk or median nerve was performed. The postoperative recovery of hand function could, therefore, only be attributed to the nerve reconstruction.[57] The analysis of our surgical results showed that useful reanimation of the hand was obtained in 69% of patients (Raimondi score ≥3).[68] Only a few other reports concerning recovery of hand function were published. Haerle and Gilbert[77] reported 76% good recovery of hand function, but in this series, secondary surgery (ie, tendon transfers) had also been performed on several patients. In Birch and colleagues'[35] series of 47 patients, 57% regained a Raimondi score greater than or equal to 4 and 93% regained a Raimondi score greater than or equal to 3.

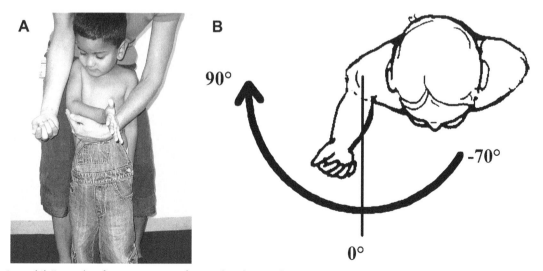

Fig. 8. (*A*) Example of measurement of true glenohumeral external rotation in adduction; trick movements are eliminated. Note the extended wrist to compensate for a lack of external rotation. (*B*) Measurement angle of external rotation.

SUMMARY

An OBPL is not an uncommon birth injury; 20% to 30% of infants who have this condition may have incomplete spontaneous recovery. As a consequence, functional disability remains, which might affect their upper limb function for the rest of their lives. The level of functional loss depends on the extent of the nerve lesion. Selection for appropriate surgical treatment is challenging and requires experience, as does the nerve reconstructive surgery. Good results with nerve reconstructive surgery have been obtained, significantly improving the functionality of the arm to a level that would probably not have been reached through spontaneous regeneration and conservative treatment. Specialized centers with a multidisciplinary approach are probably best suited for the treatment of these infants.

REFERENCES

1. Clark LP, Taylor AS, Prout TP. A study on brachial birth palsy. Am J Med Sci 1905;130(4):670–705.
2. Metaizeau JP, Gayet C, Plenat F. [Brachial plexus birth injuries. An experimental study] [in French]. Chir Pediatr 1979;20(3):159–63.
3. Bager B. Perinatally acquired brachial plexus palsy– a persisting challenge. Acta Paediatr 1997;86(11): 1214–9.
4. Dawodu A, Sankaran-Kutty M, Rajan TV. Risk factors and prognosis for brachial plexus injury and clavicular fracture in neonates: a prospective analysis from the United Arab Emirates. Ann Trop Paediatr 1997;17(3):195–200.
5. Evans-Jones G, Kay SP, Weindling AM, et al. Congenital brachial palsy: incidence, causes, and outcome in the United Kingdom and Republic of Ireland. Arch Dis Child Fetal Neonatal Ed 2003; 88(3):F185–9.
6. Gilbert WM, Nesbitt TS, Danielsen B. Associated factors in 1611 cases of brachial plexus injury. Obstet Gynecol 1999;93(4):536–40.
7. Levine MG, Holroyde J, Woods JR, et al. Birth trauma: incidence and predisposing factors. Obstet Gynecol 1984;63(6):792–5.
8. Geutjens G, Gilbert A, Helsen K. Obstetric brachial plexus palsy associated with breech delivery. A different pattern of injury. J Bone Joint Surg Br 1996;78(2):303–6.
9. Gurewitsch ED, Allen RH. Shoulder dystocia. Clin Perinatol 2007;34(3):365–85.
10. Lerner HM, Salamon E. Permanent brachial plexus injury following vaginal delivery without physician traction or shoulder dystocia. Am J Obstet Gynecol 2008;198(3):e7–8.
11. Jacobsen S. [Occurrence of obstetrical injuries to the brachial plexus on the islands of Lolland and Falster 1960–1970] [in Danish]. Nord Med 1971; 86(42):1200–1.
12. Sjoberg I, Erichs K, Bjerre I. Cause and effect of obstetric (neonatal) brachial plexus palsy. Acta Paediatr Scand 1988;77(3):357–64.
13. Al Qattan MM, Clarke HM, Curtis CG. Klumpke's birth palsy. Does it really exist? J Hand Surg [Br] 1995;20(1):19–23.
14. Sunderland S. Nerve injuries and their repair: a critical appraisal. Edingburgh, London, Melbourne. New York: Churchill Livingstone; 1991.
15. Adler JB, Patterson RL. Erb's palsy. Long-term results of treatment in eighty-eight cases. J Bone Joint Surg Am 1967;49(6):1052–64.
16. Bellew M, Kay SP, Webb F, et al. Developmental and behavioural outcome in obstetric brachial plexus palsy. J Hand Surg Br 2000;25(1):49–51.
17. Gjorup L. Obstetrical lesion of the brachial plexus. Acta Neurol Scand 1966;42(Suppl):1–80.
18. Pearl ML, Edgerton BW. Glenoid deformity secondary to brachial plexus birth palsy. J Bone Joint Surg Am 1998;80(5):659–67.
19. Pollock AN, Reed MH. Shoulder deformities from obstetrical brachial plexus paralysis. Skeletal Radiol 1989;18(4):295–7.
20. Bradley WG, Daroff RB, Fenichel GM, et al. Neurology in clinical practice. 2nd edition. Boston: Butterworth-Heinemann; 1996.
21. Greenberg MS. Handbook of neurosurgery. 5th edition. New York: Thieme; 2001.
22. Laurent JP, Lee RT. Birth-related upper brachial plexus injuries in infants: operative and nonoperative approaches. J Child Neurol 1994;9(2):111–7.
23. Painter MJ, Bergman I. Obstetrical trauma to the neonatal central and peripheral nervous system. Semin Perinatol 1982;6(1):89–104.
24. Shenaq SM, Berzin E, Lee R, et al. Brachial plexus birth injuries and current management. Clin Plast Surg 1998;25(4):527–36.
25. Terzis JK, Papakonstantinou KC. Management of obstetric brachial plexus palsy. Hand Clin 1999; 15(4):717–36.
26. Gordon M, Rich H, Deutschberger J, et al. The immediate and long-term outcome of obstetric birth trauma. I. Brachial plexus paralysis. Am J Obstet Gynecol 1973;117(1):51–6.
27. Walle T, Hartikainen-Sorri AL. Obstetric shoulder injury. Associated risk factors, prediction and prognosis. Acta Obstet Gynecol Scand 1993;72(6):450–4.
28. Pondaag W, Malessy MJ, van Dijk JG, et al. Natural history of obstetric brachial plexus palsy: a systematic review. Dev Med Child Neurol 2004;46(2): 138–44.
29. Gramsbergen A, IJkema-Paassen J, Meek MF. Sciatic nerve transection in the adult rat: abnormal

EMG patterns during locomotion by aberrant innervation of hindleg muscles. Exp Neurol 2000;161(1): 183–93.

30. Roth G. [Reinnervation in obstetrical brachial plexus paralysis] [in French]. J Neurol Sci 1983;58(1): 103–15.

31. Brown T, Cupido C, Scarfone H, et al. Developmental apraxia arising from neonatal brachial plexus palsy. Neurology 2000;55(1):24–30.

32. van Dijk JG, Pondaag W, Malessy MJ. Obstetric lesions of the brachial plexus. Muscle Nerve 2001; 24(11):1451–61.

33. van Dijk JG, Pondaag W, Malessy MJ. Botulinum toxin and the pathophysiology of obstetric brachial plexus lesions [letter]. Dev Med Child Neurol 2007; 49(4):318–9.

34. Tassin JL. [Obstetric paralysis of the brachial plexus. Spontaneous recovery; results of interventions] [in French] [thesis]. Université Paris; 1983.

35. Birch R, Ahad N, Kono H, et al. Repair of obstetric brachial plexus palsy: results in 100 children. J Bone Joint Surg Br 2005;87(8):1089–95.

36. Clarke HM, Al Qattan MM, Curtis CG, et al. Obstetrical brachial plexus palsy: results following neurolysis of conducting neuromas-in-continuity. Plast Reconstr Surg 1996;97(5):974–82.

37. Gilbert A, Tassin JL. [Surgical repair of the brachial plexus in obstetric paralysis] [in French]. Chirurgie 1984;110(1):70–5.

38. Kawabata H, Masada K, Tsuyuguchi Y, et al. Early microsurgical reconstruction in birth palsy. Clin Orthop Relat Res 1987;(215):233–42.

39. Waters PM. Update on management of pediatric brachial plexus palsy. J Pediatr Orthop B 2005; 14(4):233–44.

40. Michelow BJ, Clarke HM, Curtis CG, et al. The natural history of obstetrical brachial plexus palsy. Plast Reconstr Surg 1994;93(4):675–80.

41. Smith NC, Rowan P, Benson LJ, et al. Neonatal brachial plexus palsy. Outcome of absent biceps function at three months of age. J Bone Joint Surg Am 2004;86-A(10):2163–70.

42. Waters PM. Comparison of the natural history, the outcome of microsurgical repair, and the outcome of operative reconstruction in brachial plexus birth palsy. J Bone Joint Surg Am 1999;81(5):649–59.

43. Fisher DM, Borschel GH, Curtis CG, et al. Evaluation of elbow flexion as a predictor of outcome in obstetrical brachial plexus palsy. Plast Reconstr Surg 2007;120(6):1585–90.

44. Borrero JL, de Pawlikowski W. Obstetrical brachial plexus palsy. Lima (Peru): MAD Corp S.A; 2005.

45. Clarke HM, Curtis CG. An approach to obstetrical brachial plexus injuries. Hand Clin 1995;11(4):563–80.

46. Bisinella GL, Birch R, Smith SJ. Neurophysiological prediction of outcome in obstetric lesions of the brachial plexus. J Hand Surg Br 2003;28(2):148–52.

47. Bellew M, Kay SP. Early parental experiences of obstetric brachial plexus palsy. J Hand Surg Br 2003;28(4):339–46.

48. van Dijk JG, Malessy MJ, Stegeman DF. Why is the electromyogram in obstetric brachial plexus lesions overly optimistic? [letter]. Muscle Nerve 1998;21(2): 260–1.

49. Vredeveld JW, Blaauw G, Slooff BA, et al. The findings in paediatric obstetric brachial palsy differ from those in older patients: a suggested explanation. Dev Med Child Neurol 2000;42(3):158–61.

50. Zalis OS, Zalis AW, Barron KD, et al. Motor patterning following transitory sensory-motor deprivations. Arch Neurol 1965;13(5):487–94.

51. Grossman JA. Early operative intervention for birth injuries to the brachial plexus. Semin Pediatr Neurol 2000;7(1):36–43.

52. American Society for Peripheral Nerve. Presented at the Annual Scientific Meeting. Rio Grande, Puerto Rico, January 13–14, 2007.

53. Xu J, Cheng X, Gu Y. Different methods and results in the treatment of obstetrical brachial plexus palsy. J Reconstr Microsurg 2000;16(6):417–20.

54. Kline DG. Different methods and results in the treatment of obstetrical brachial plexus palsy [letter]. J Reconstr Microsurg 2000;16(6):420–2.

55. Bodensteiner JB, Rich KM, Landau WM. Early infantile surgery for birth-related brachial plexus injuries: justification requires a prospective controlled study. J Child Neurol 1994;9(2):109–10.

56. Kay SP. Obstetrical brachial palsy. Br J Plast Surg 1998;51(1):43–50.

57. Pondaag W, Malessy MJ. Recovery of hand function following nerve grafting and transfer in obstetric brachial plexus lesions. J Neurosurg (1 Suppl Pediatrics) 2006;105(1 Suppl):33–40.

58. Walker AT, Chaloupka JC, de Lotbiniere AC, et al. Detection of nerve rootlet avulsion on CT myelography in patients with birth palsy and brachial plexus injury after trauma. AJR Am J Roentgenol 1996; 167(5):1283–7.

59. Chow BC, Blaser S, Clarke HM. Predictive value of computed tomographic myelography in obstetrical brachial plexus palsy. Plast Reconstr Surg 2000; 106(5):971–7.

60. Aszmann OC, Rab M, Kamolz L, et al. The anatomy of the pectoral nerves and their significance in brachial plexus reconstruction. J Hand Surg [Am] 2000;25(5):942–7.

61. Malessy MJ, Thomeer RT. Evaluation of intercostal to musculocutaneous nerve transfer in reconstructive brachial plexus surgery. J Neurosurg 1998;88(2):266–71.

62. Kline DG. Nerve surgery as it is now and as it may be. Neurosurgery 2000;46(6):1285–93.

63. Tiel RL, Happel LT Jr, Kline DG. Nerve action potential recording method and equipment. Neurosurgery 1996;39(1):103–8.

64. Kline DG, Hackett ER, May PR. Evaluation of nerve injuries by evoked potentials and electromyography. J Neurosurg 1969;31(2):128–36.

65. Pondaag W, Van der Veken LPAJ, Van Someren PJ, et al. Intraoperative NAP en CMAP recordings in patients with obstetric brachial plexus lesions. J Neurosurg, in press.

66. Malessy MJ, van Duinen SG, Feirabend HK, et al. Correlation between histopathological findings in C-5 and C-6 nerve stumps and motor recovery following nerve grafting for repair of brachial plexus injury. J Neurosurg 1999;91(4):636–44.

67. Mallet J. [Obstetrical paralysis of the brachial plexus. II. Therapeutics. Treatment of sequelae. Priority for the treatment of the shoulder. Method for the expression of results] [in French]. Rev Chir Orthop Reparatrice Appar Mot 1972;58(Suppl 1):166–8.

68. Raimondi P. Evaluation of results in obstetric brachial plexus palsy. The hand. Presented at the International Meeting on Obstetric Brachial Plexus Palsy. Heerlen, The Netherlands, 1993.

69. Gilbert A, Brockman R, Carlioz H. Surgical treatment of brachial plexus birth palsy. Clin Orthop 1991;264: 39–47.

70. Laurent JP, Lee R, Shenaq S, et al. Neurosurgical correction of upper brachial plexus birth injuries. J Neurosurg 1993;79(2):197–203.

71. Pondaag W, de BR, Van Wijlen-Hempel MS, et al. External rotation as a result of suprascapular nerve neurotization in obstetric brachial plexus lesions. Neurosurgery 2005;57(3):530–7.

72. Kawabata H, Shibata T, Matsui Y, et al. Use of intercostal nerves for neurotization of the musculocutaneous nerve in infants with birth-related brachial plexus palsy. J Neurosurg 2001;94(3):386–91.

73. Blaauw G, Slooff AC. Transfer of pectoral nerves to the musculocutaneous nerve in obstetric upper brachial plexus palsy. Neurosurgery 2003;53(2): 338–41.

74. Al Qattan MM. Oberlin's ulnar nerve transfer to the biceps nerve in Erb's birth palsy [letter]. Plast Reconstr Surg 2002;109(1):405–7.

75. Noaman HH, Shiha AE, Bahm J. Oberlin's ulnar nerve transfer to the biceps motor nerve in obstetric brachial plexus palsy: indications, and good and bad results. Microsurgery 2004;24(3):182–7.

76. Narakas AO, Allieu Y, Alnot JY, et al. [Complete supraclavicular paralysis. Surgical possibilities and results] [in French]. In: Alnot JY, Narakas AO, editors. [Paralysis of the brachial plexus]. Paris: Expansion Scientifique Francaise; 1989. p. 130–62.

77. Haerle M, Gilbert A. Management of complete obstetric brachial plexus lesions. J Pediatr Orthop 2004;24(2):194–200.

Brachial Plexus Injury: The London Experience with Supraclavicular Traction Lesions

Rolfe Birch, MChir, FRCS&P (Glas), FRCS (Edin), FRCS (Eng)

KEYWORDS
- Brachial plexus injuries • Neuropathic pain
- Timing of repair

George Bonney introduced a policy of urgent repair of injuries to main nerves in the early 1960s at St Mary's Hospital, London. The case was considered an emergency if the nerve injury was complicated by a rupture of a main artery at the same site. This policy was extended to the closed supraclavicular lesion, and the first urgent repair was performed in 1962. Other repairs had been done earlier, in selected cases, at the Royal National Orthopaedic Hospital (**Fig. 1**). The results of grafting of the ruptured spinal nerves were generally poor, which, with the high incidence of preganglionic (avulsion) lesions, was disappointing. Several operations were performed for the purpose of establishing diagnosis alone. It was the work of his friend, Algimantas Narakas, of Lausanne, which stimulated Bonney to make a fresh start in 1974. The results in 1162 operations for supraclavicular injuries were outlined in 1998.[1] In all, repairs by one means or another have been performed in more than 1500 cases of the closed traction lesion in the adult since 1962.

Important advances have been made in methods of diagnosis and repair during this time. Myelography[2] was replaced at St Mary's Hospital by CT scan with contrast enhancement[3] and later by MRI. The early work of Bonney[4] and of Bonney and Gilliatt[5] was extended to the analysis of central conduction by Landi and colleagues[6] in 1980 at the Royal National Orthopaedic Hospital and this seminal work has become a central, essential component in the diagnosis of lesions exposed within a few days of injury.

New methods of repair were introduced. The free vascularized ulnar nerve graft was introduced by Jamieson with Bonney in 1975.[7] The first repair of the intradural lesion was carried out by Bonney and Jamieson in 1977 in one case operated within 24 hours of injury.

With the patient in the left lateral position, I exposed the brachial plexus above the clavicle; the plexus had, as was expected, been completely avulsed. I marked the 7th and 8th cervical nerves and their roots. I then exposed the posterior elements of the cervical spine through a posterior incision, and went onto expose the right side of the cervical dura by hemi laminectomy. I opened the dura to expose the right side of the spinal cord and to show the

Royal National Orthopaedic Hospital, 6 Hill House, 173 Stanmore Hill, Stanmore H37 3EW, UK
E-mail address: benita.patel@rnoh.nhs.uk

Neurosurg Clin N Am 20 (2009) 15–23
doi:10.1016/j.nec.2008.08.002
1042-3680/08/$ – see front matter © 2008 Published by Elsevier Inc.

neurosurgery.theclinics.com

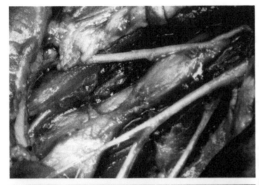
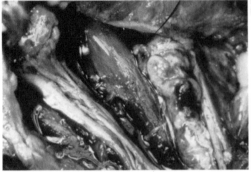

Fig. 1. Repair by graft of lesion of upper trunk of the brachial plexus using fibrin clot glue. (*Courtesy of George Bonney and Donal Brooks. Royal National Orthopaedic Hospital, 1952.*)

avulsion of the roots. Now, I passed fine forceps through the foramina between the 6th and 7th and 7th and 8th vertebrae, and with these caught hold of sutures tied to the cuffs of dura at the junction of roots with peripheral nerves. With these sutures, the roots were drawn back into the spinal canal. Forceful traction was not needed; the roots lay easily in the canal, offering themselves for re-attachment.[8]

The rupture had taken place just distal to the surface of the cord; little stumps of the rootlets were visible and Jamieson sutured the dorsal rootlets of the two nerves. I reviewed this patient 10 years later. He was well adjusted, in full-time work, and had no pain. He demonstrated remarkable recovery into pectoralis major and biceps muscles, which perhaps confirms Carlstedt's[9] view that the ventral neurone can find its way out to the periphery through a pathway between the spinal cord and the avulsed spinal nerve.

Advice and examples from such friends and colleagues as Aligimantas Narakas, Yves Allieu, Laurent Sedel, Christophe Oberlin, Alain Gilbert, and Akira Nagano led to the extensive use of nerve transfers from 1980.

The incidence of this injury was described by Goldie and Coates,[10] who wrote to every

orthopedic surgeon and to other interested surgeons in the United Kingdom. Details of 328 cases of injuries to the supraclavicular plexus were analyzed. The lesion was complete in 22.8%. A wound existed in 5.1%. The subclavian artery was ruptured in 4.7% and no less than 43% of these patients had other major injuries. It seems that the severity of the lesion is declining (**Table 1**).

THE LESION

The level of lesion has been clarified. The observation of small stumps of the dorsal rootlets led to the idea that the preganglionic injury should be considered as either central to the transitional zone or peripheral to it. Schenker[11] examined the tips of the roots of avulsed spinal nerves and found that most of these were torn peripheral to the transitional zone.[12] Schenker[13] also confirmed that the ventral root in man contains myelinated afferent fibers. This fact may be relevant in the relief of pain by reinnervation of skeletal muscle and it may also underlie the absence of cocontraction, which is seen in many cases of selective reinnervation of the avulsed ventral root.

INDICATIONS FOR URGENT EXPLORATION

Magalon and colleagues[14] set out the case clearly: "It is advisable because emergency nerve surgery is technically easier and because the overall results are better if combined vascular and nerve injuries are involved immediate emergency surgery is mandatory." These workers also provide good advice in situations where only the great vessels can be repaired: "Positioning ruptured nerves away from the vascular bypass will greatly facilitate second stage repair." The biologic imperative for repair of ruptured nerves as soon as possible is established beyond any reasonable doubt and is supported by numerous clinical studies. The last 25 years have seen a growing appreciation of the central effects of proximal axonotomy.[15,16] The central response is swift and occurs within hours or minutes.[17,18] I have come to the view that repair in the closed traction lesion comes, in urgency, close behind reattachment of the amputated hand or repair of a great artery and a trunk nerve in the combined lesion, and it is a pleasing duty to acknowledge the clinical acumen of so many of our colleagues, mostly orthopedic surgeons, throughout the United Kingdom who have made it possible for us to do this work by virtue of their early recognition of the severity of the injury and by their appreciation that it may, in fact, be possible to do something useful for the patient.

Table 1
The changing lesion displayed at operation: samples of 40 years of experience

Years	Total Number of Patients	Total Number of Spinal Nerves	Nerves Avulsed	Avulsion C5–T1	Arterial Injury
1966–1984	210	1100	690 (63%)	48 (23%)	26 (12%)
1989–1993	300 (consecutive)	1500	826 (55%)	52 (17%)	21 (7%)
2003–2006	320 (consecutive)	1600	730 (46%)	26 (8%)	16 (5%)

DIAGNOSIS

The history is all important. The direction of application of force and some understanding of the violence of that force comes first. Deep bruising indicates tearing of deep structures; ecchymosis or abrasions over the neck and the shoulder show the application of force. Sensory loss involving the cervical plexus suggests serious injury to the upper spinal nerves (**Fig. 2**). Two other features are important. The first is pain. Nearly one half of our patients have been seen within the first week or two of injury, and most describe immediate onset of pain, or its development, within 24 hours. The pain was eloquently described by Frazier and Skillern's[19] patient in 1911:

The pain is continuous, it does not stop for a minute either day or night. It is either burning or compressing… ….. in addition there is, every few minutes, a jerking sensation similar to that …… by clutching….. a Leyden jar. It is like a zig zag made in the sky by a stroke of lightening. The upper part of the arm is mostly free of pain; the lower part from a little above the elbow to the tips of the fingers, never.[19]

It is all here. The pain is severe, it has two parts (one constant, the other intermittent), and it is worst in the hand and forearm. The lightning pain is usually expressed within the first 24 or 48 hours after injury and it is precisely distributed. If it radiates to the radial aspect of the forearm and the thumb, then avulsion of C6 is likely. If it radiates to the back of the hand, then a similar lesion is likely at C7. When it radiates down the inner side of the forearm and into the fingers, then the lowest nerves are similarly damaged.

The second factor is the presence or absence of the Tinel sign, which is detectable on the day of injury in postganglionic rupture, and the irradiation of pins and needles advises the clinician which spinal nerves have been ruptured.[20] For C5, irradiation is to the elbow; for C6, it is to the radial aspect of the forearm and the base of the thumb, and for C7, it is to the back of the hand. We have recently examined the validity of this finding in 300 consecutive operated cases and found that the prediction of rupture was confirmed in close to 90% of the spinal nerves so diagnosed.

Examination of the extent of paralysis is important, paying particular attention to serratus anterior and trapezius muscles and to the ipsilateral hemidiaphragm. The evidence provided by the history and by clinical examination should enable the clinician to make accurate diagnosis of the extent and depth of injury and to form a fairly clear idea of the level of lesion. That diagnosis is clarified by CT scan with contrast enhancement or by MRI and it is finally established at operation.

These injuries are high energy transfer injuries. In at least 15% of our patients, other potentially life-threatening injuries, which must take absolute priority, have enforced delay. Care must be taken to seek out occult injury to the spinal cord, the spinal column, the chest, and the abdominal viscera at the receiving hospital and again at the hospital to which that patient is transferred. The treatment of significant injuries to the head, to the spinal column and chest, and to the abdomen and pelvis come first.

INTRAOPERATIVE STUDY OF CONDUCTION

The study of somatosensory evoked potentials from the proximal stump of ruptured nerves enables recognition of the combined partial avulsion complicating distal rupture and it also points to selective injury to either the ventral or the dorsal root. Placing grafts onto a stump where central conduction is abnormal or absent is usually fruitless (**Fig. 3**). Analysis of distal conduction in urgent cases is informative; it is usually present for up to 80 hours after injury. In one case, distal conduction in the avulsed ventral root was present at 132 hours after injury.

The patient illustrated in **Fig. 4** came off his motorcycle at speed on the day before Christmas Eve. The referring surgeon diagnosed rupture of the subclavian artery, so providing the opportunity

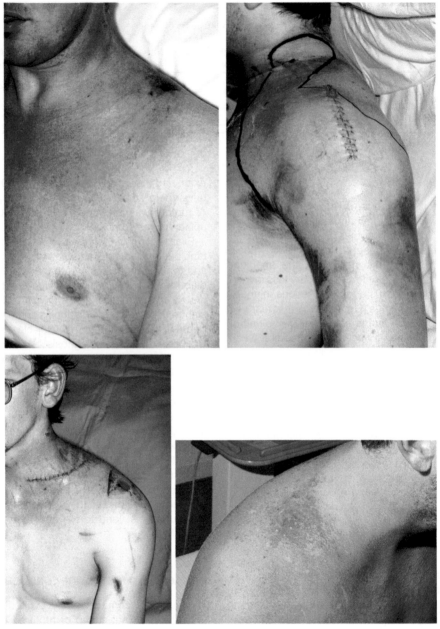

Fig. 2. Some examples of bruising, abrasion, and extensive sensory loss, which indicate extent and severity of injury.

to deal with this at the same time as dealing with the nerve injury in a limb, which was not critically ischemic. Operation was undertaken at 60 hours. The clinical diagnosis was confirmed. Postganglionic rupture of C5 and of C6, with avulsion of C7, C8, and T1, was easily demonstrated. Stimulation of the avulsed ventral roots was followed by the appropriate response in distal muscles, which showed us three things. First, that critical ischemia of muscle or nerve had not occurred; next, that a second injury to any major nerve trunk had not occurred; and finally, that we could confine resection of the tips of the ventral roots to no more than a millimeter or two. This case illustrates the technical ease of early exposure and how easy it is to diminish the gap between the stumps. The avulsed spinal nerves had been pulled downwards to lie below the clavicle.

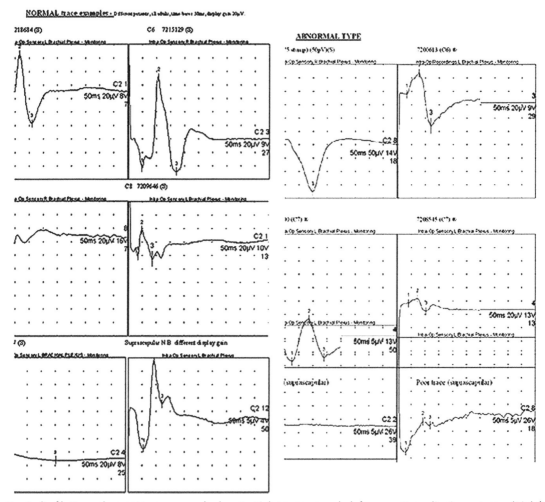

Fig. 3. (*Left*) Normal somatosensory evoked potential traces recorded from postganglionic ruptures. (*Right*) Abnormal traces recorded from postganglionic ruptures indicate an element of preganglionic injury.

PRINCIPLES OF REPAIR

The closed traction lesion falls into one of two broad groups. In the first, which accounts for nearly one half of our cases, a lower nerve is intact or recovering and the upper nerves have been damaged. The patient has the potential for hand function, and the object of restoration of function at shoulder and elbow can usually be achieved. It should be the rule that a useful and relatively pain-free limb is achieved by combining graft with specific nerve transfer, and by transfer of

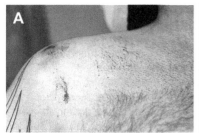
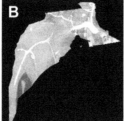
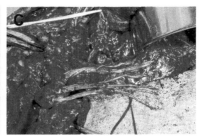

Fig. 4. (A) Soft tissue abrasions around the shoulder and neck with pain with percussion into the C5 and C6 distributions suggested postganglionic ruptures of these elements. (B) Conventional angiogram demonstrates subclavian artery occlusion. (C) Operative appearance of the preganglionic lesions to C7, C8, and T1.

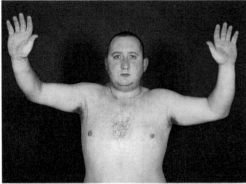

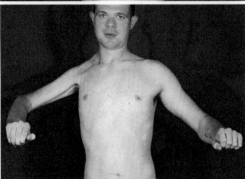

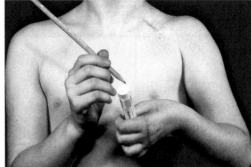

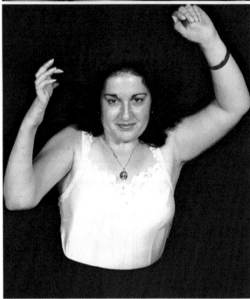

Fig. 5. (*Top*) A 23-year-old manual laborer who sustained rupture of C5 with avulsion of C6 and C7, with recovery for C8 and T1. Repair at 3 days was done by graft and nerve transfers. The spinal accessory nerve was transferred to the ventral root of C7. He considered function within his limb as normal at 24 months. In this case, reinnervation of the ventral root of C7 restored function in triceps and in the wrist extensor muscles (*Bottom*). A 24-year-old electrician who sustained rupture of C5, avulsion of C6, C7, C8, with recovery of T1. Repair was done by graft and by nerve transfers. The spinal accessory nerve was transferred to the ventral root of C6. The operation was done at 4 days after injury. At 9 months, a successful flexor-to-extensor transfer was done. His function was good enough for him to be able to return to his trade. In both patients, pain was severe for the first 9 months after operation. It resolved with return of muscle function.

Fig. 6. Elements of hand function were regained in both of these patients who sustained postganglionic rupture of C5, C6, and C7, with avulsion of C8 and T1. (*Top*) A 7-year-old child who was operated 8 weeks after injury at age 3. (*Bottom*) A 17-year-old woman 3 years after repair, which was done at 6 days from injury.

the spinal accessory nerve to either the suprascapular nerve or the avulsed ventral root, with timely musculotendinous transfer (**Fig. 5**).

In the complete lesion, every reasonable effort should be made to display postganglionic ruptures. The finding of even one rupture makes a great deal of difference. In earlier years, we hoped that the free vascularized ulnar nerve graft would not only regain elbow flexion but also restore hand function by reinnervation of the median nerve (**Fig. 6**).[1,7] Only 14 of 65 patients regained wrist and finger flexion to the Medical Research Council 3 or better, with sensory recovery to light touch, pin prick, and warm sense within the median territory. In 13 of these cases, the operation was done within 14 days of injury. Useful hand function was regained in only 3 patients. Pain persisted in some patients despite recovery of function. We abandoned the method about 15 years ago, preferring instead to repair the whole of the plexus in cases that involve two or three postganglionic ruptures with avulsion of the remainder.

Recovery after repair of the spinal nerves of the brachial plexus is determined by several factors. Among these, delay before repair and the severity of the injury come first. **Table 2** outlines the results of 37 spinal nerves repaired by either graft or nerve transfer in 153 cases operated in the years 1991 to 1993. One third of patients achieved no useful

Table 2
Recovery by delay and severity of lesion: 367 spinal nerves repaired by graft or by transfer in 153 cases operated during 1991 to 1993

	Interval from Injury to Repair			
Recovery	Within 14 Days	To 3 Months	To 6 Months	To 12 Months
Partial lesion (at least one intact nerve, usually C8 or T1)				
Useful	75	83	16	11
Failure	11	25	3	11
Complete lesion (mixed rupture and avulsion C5–T1)				
Useful	43	15	3	7
Failure	22	17	6	19

These figures exclude repairs using the vascularized ulnar nerve graft and also intercostal transfers for pain relief, hand sensation, and medial cord function.

function. Forty-three cases achieved good function across two joints in the upper limb and, of these, 33 were operated within 14 days of injury. Four patients regained useful hand function following repair of the whole of the plexus. All four were operated within 14 days.

A more recent study comes from Kato,[21] who studied the effects of operative delay on the relief of neuropathic pain in 148 patients in whom at least one spinal nerve was avulsed. The average number of avulsed spinal nerves in this series was 3.2. In 80 patients, pain was apparent at the moment of injury or within 24 hours, and it developed within 2 weeks in 35 more. In 15 cases, intubation and ventilation was necessary for up to 3 weeks and for these, recollection of the onset of pain was difficult. All patients experienced severe pain that was slightly worse where the lower roots were avulsed. Kato divided his patients into four groups based on the interval between injury and exploration: group 1 (early), within 1 month of injury (n = 61); group 2 (delayed), 1 to 3 months after injury (n = 29); group 3 (late), 3 to 6 months after injury (n = 32); group 4 (neglected), more than 6 months after in jury (n = 26). Results were decisively better in the early group. Recovery of function and relief of pain were strongly correlated.

It is tempting to suggest that the improvement in pain so often seen with reinnervation of muscle is brought about by restoration of the deep afferent pathway from muscle.[22] However, late intercostal nerve transfer is sometimes effective for the relief of pain, even when functional recovery of skeletal muscle is not a realistic prospect.[23] Several explanations are possible. First, the transfer of healthy intercostal nerves into the trunk nerves of the upper limb may inhibit abnormal electric activity within the substantia gelatinosa. Second, relief from pain may purely be a nonspecific effect of

operation, depending on the anesthetic used, the degree of postoperative pain, and the use of analgesics, or on suggestion alone. Third, relief may be produced by sectioning functioning axons of the posterior root system, impulses from which have, in some way, been reaching the central nervous system. However, as Kato[19] pointed out, a few of the patients in his series showed a dramatic improvement in their neuropathic pain immediately after operation, whereas others showed relief from pain shortly after their return to work, suggesting that psychologic factors are important.

THE COMPLETE PREGANGLIONIC INJURY: AVULSION C5 TO T1

Carlstedt has continued and expanded work towards reconnecting the spinal cord to avulsed spinal nerves and more than 30 cases have been done at the Royal National Orthopaedic Hospital since 1996. Some remarkable results have followed. That regeneration from the spinal cord into the peripheral nervous system does occur is no longer a question for debate: what is required is refinement in selection, in appreciation of risk, and improvement in technique. Flow through the anterior spinal artery is maintained by radicular vessels concentrated at the cervical and lumbar enlargements.[24,25] An incomplete Brown-Séquard syndrome is detectable in at least 10% of cases of complete avulsion. Diminution of flow through the anterior spinal artery caused by interruption of the radicular arteries is one possible explanation. Potential ischemia of the cervical cord overshadows attempts at reimplantation of avulsed spinal nerves. Direct access to the ruptured ventral root is an interesting possibility. In one of our cases, a small joint arthroscope introduced into the foramen of C8 revealed the ventral root floating around in the

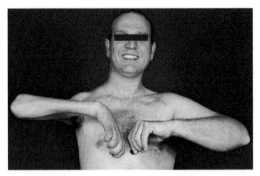

Fig. 7. "Distraction or destruction." This 44-year-old man sustained avulsion of C6, C7, C8 and T1, with severe lesion of C5. We repaired the subclavian artery on the day of injury but no repair of the nerves was possible. He had useful spontaneous recovery into the suprascapular nerve and a successful free muscle transfer (latissimus dorsi) restored elbow flexion. He returned to full-time work 3 months after his injury because it helped his pain. The motto is his.

cerebrospinal fluid, and in three cases it was possible to graft onto the stump of the ventral root. Such cases offer a challenge for future development.

SUMMARY

To the biologic imperative of urgency of repair in these severe injuries is added the technical ease of early exploration. We have dismal experience of operations in late cases, where fibrosis prevented full analysis of the lesion and restricted opportunities for repair. In some cases, fibrosis was so severe that the operation was abandoned, which was particularly true where undue delay occurred between emergency repair of subclavian artery and exploration of the nerve lesion. Some methods of repair are possible only in the early days after injury, and these include selective reinnervation of the ventral root and reattachment of the avulsed spinal nerves to the spinal cord. The gap between stumps can be greatly diminished and, often, the distal stumps lie deep to, or even below, the clavicle. Recording of central conduction is essential in the analysis of the lesion in early cases to ascertain the quality of the proximal stump.

The traction lesion of the supraclavicular brachial plexus is different from that seen involving the cords of the brachial plexus in a severe infraclavicular lesion where nerves may be greatly stretched but not ruptured, presenting a difficult problem for the operating surgeon. Instead, the injury to the spinal nerve in the posterior triangle is clearly one of avulsion, rupture, or recovery. Preparation of the stumps of the damaged nerves is much easier in the early cases, especially when peripheral conduction is still present. Resection back to a recognizable architecture usually coincides with return of conduction centrally and distally and it is remarkable how little we resect. I reject the idea that early repair will be compromised by fibrosis; the most difficult and the most fruitless cases that we have encountered have been sent to us late.

Associated injuries, and injuries to the spinal cord and the spinal column, can impose an absolute contraindication to urgent exploration of the brachial plexus in at least 15% of all of our cases. The risk for a gush of cerebrospinal fluid is also a factor in the early case. Although we have never experienced a case of coning, the clinician responsible must bear the possibility in mind, and sealing of the dural tear by absorbable sponge, fibrin clot glue, and plugs of muscle or fat is necessary.

The object of operation in the incomplete case, in those patients in whom C8 and T1 have survived, is to restore useful function to the upper limb by reinnervation of the shoulder and elbow. No muscle transfer at the shoulder girdle or elbow ever matches the results seen after a good nerve repair. Early improvement of hand function by musculotendinous transfer is facilitated by clear knowledge of the prognosis for the nerves.

In the complete lesion, the object of operation is to reinnervate two segments, or even more, within the limb, and one of the major aims of reinnervation is to ease pain. Complete avulsion is a terrible injury and much more work needs to be done to explore the opportunities for reconnection between the spinal cord and the peripheral nervous system set out by the pioneering work of George Bonney and Thomas Carlstedt. The clinician should never forget that the patient who has a complete lesion of the brachial plexus will endure misery and depression for many months. His/her livelihood is threatened. The operation is but the first step in rehabilitation. The first surgeon must actively engage in the whole process of rehabilitation, and must engage him/herself in active treatment of pain, in the mitigation of disability by provision of orthoses, and in actively supporting early return to work, return to work modified, early training for alternative work, or return to study. These patients need to be followed for many years and the later development of neurologic symptoms or worsening of pain requires thorough investigation.

Most of these patients are risk takers, and most demonstrate remarkable spirit and fortitude. Their loyal appreciation of efforts, which are all too often unavailing, is most rewarding (**Fig. 7**).

REFERENCES

1. Birch R. Traumatic lesions of the brachial plexus. In: Birch R, Bonney G, Wynn Parry CB, editors. Surgical disorders of the peripheral nerves. Edinburgh (UK): Churchill Livingstone London; 1998. p. 157–208.
2. Davis ER, Sutton D, Bligh AS. Myelography in brachial plexus injury. Br J Radiol 1966;39:362–71.
3. Marshall RW, de SILVA RD. Computerised tomography in traction lesions of the brachial plexus. J Bone Joint Surg Br 1986;68:734–8.
4. Bonney G. The value of axon responses in determining the site of lesion in traction lesions of the brachial plexus. Brain 1954;77:588–609.
5. Bonney G, Gilliatt RW. Sensory nerve conduction after traction lesion of the brachial plexus. Proc R Soc Med 1958;51:365–7.
6. Landi A, Copeland SA, Wynn-Parry CB, et al. The role of somatosensory evoked potentials and nerve conduction studies in the surgical management of brachial plexus injuries. J Bone Joint Surg Br 1980;62:492–6.
7. Birch R, Dunkerton M, Bonney G, et al. Experience with the free vascularised ulnar nerve graft in repair of supraclavicular lesion of the brachial plexus. Clin Orthop Relat Res 1988;237:96–104.
8. Bonney G. Reimplantation of avulsed spinal nerves. The first clinical case. In: Birch R, Bonney G, Wynn Parry CB, editors. Surgical disorders of the peripheral nerves. 1st edition. London: Churchill Livingstone; 1998. p. 200–2.
9. Carlstedt T, Crane P, Hallin RG, et al. Return of function after spinal cord implantation of avulsed spinal nerve roots. Lancet 1995;346:1323–5.
10. Goldie BS, Coates CJ. Brachial plexus injuries– a survey of incidence and referral pattern. J Hand Surg [Br] 1992;17:86–8.
11. Schenker M. Analysis of avulsed roots in traction injury of the human brachial plexus. Thesis for MSc in Surgical Science, University College of London, 1998.
12. Schenker M, Birch R. Diagnosis of level of intradural ruptures of the rootlets in traction lesions of the brachial plexus. J Bone Joint Surg Br 2001;83:916–20.
13. Schenker M, Birch R. Intact myelinated fibres in biopsies of ventral spinal roots after preganglionic traction injury to the brachial plexus. A proof that Sherrington's "wrong way afferents" exist in man? J Anat 2000;197:383–91.
14. Magalon G, Bordeaux J, Legree R, et al. Emergency versus delayed repair of severe brachial plexus injuries. Clin Orthop Relat Res 1988;237:32–6.
15. Dyck PJ, Nukada H, Lais CA, et al. Permanent axotomy: a model of chronic neuronal degeneration produced by axonal atrophy, myelin remodelling and regeneration. In: Dyck PJ, Thomas PK, Lambert EH, Bunge R, editors. Peripheral neuropathy. 2nd edition. Philadelphia: W B Saunders; 1984. p. 660–90.
16. Groves MJ, Scaravilli F. Pathology of peripheral neurone cell bodies. In: Dyke PJ, Thomas PK, editors. Peripheral neuropathy. 4th edition. Philadelphia: Elsevier Saunders; 2005. p. 683–732, Chapter 31.
17. Lawson SN. The peripheral sensory nervous system: dorsal root ganglion neurones. In: Dyck PJ, Thomas PK, editors. Peripheral neuropathy (in two volumes). 4th edition. Philadelphia: Elsevier Saunders; 2005. p. 163–202, Chapter 8.
18. Rabert D, Xiao Y, Yiangou Y, et al. Plasticity of gene expression in injured human dorsal root ganglia revealed by gene chip oligonucleotide microarrays. J Clin Neurosci 2004;11:289–99.
19. Frazier CH, Skillern PG. Supraclavicular subcutaneous lesions of the brachial plexus not associated with skeletal injuries. JAMA 1911;57:1957–63.
20. Landi A, Copeland S. Value of the Tinel sign in brachial plexus lesions. Ann R Coll Surg Engl 1979;61:470–1.
21. Kato N, Htut M, Taggart M, et al. The effects of operative delay on the relief of neuropathic pain after injury to the brachial plexus. J Bone Joint Surg Br 2006;88:756–9.
22. Berman JS, Birch R, Anand P. Pain following human brachial plexus injury with spinal cord root avulsion and the effect of surgery. Pain 1998;75:199–207.
23. Berman J, Anand P, Chen L, et al. Pain relief from preganglionic injury to the brachial plexus by late intercostal transfer. J Bone Joint Surg 1996;78B:759–60.
24. Dommisse GF. The arteries and veins of the human spinal cord from birth. 1st edition. Edinburgh (UK): Churchill Livingstone; 1975.
25. Dommisse GF. The blood supply of the spinal cord. A critical vascular zone in spinal surgery. J Bone Joint Surg Br 1974;56:225–35.

Timing for Brachial Plexus Injury: A Personal Experience

David G. Kline, MD[a,b]

KEYWORDS

• Timing • Brachial plexus injury • Electrophysiologic studies

The editors have requested the author's personal views on the timing of surgery for nerve injury and especially that for brachial plexus injuries. Although the author appreciates the experimental data and less frequent clinical outcomes suggesting that early repair gives better results than delayed repair, there are other considerations that may favor a more measured approach for repair. The following observations are personal and based on the author's own experience; thus, they must be read or viewed in that context.

The mechanism of injury producing the plexopathy is important, because some injuries have the potential for recovery, whereas others are less likely to recover on their own. Early surgery on all, especially if suture or graft repairs are done, might preclude spontaneous recovery, which, in the author's experience, almost always exceeds, when graded properly, what can be gained by repair. Conversely, neglect of repair or greatly delayed repair is equally deleterious, because, many useful outcomes can now be gained by nerve repair or transfer.

INDICATIONS FOR ACUTE REPAIR
Associated Vascular Lesions

Expanding clot, arteriovenous (A-V) fistula, and pseudoaneurysm can convert a partial injury to a more complete one and require attention in the early hours or on the first or second day after injury or shortly after the diagnosis or suspicion of such.

Decompression of the plexus and repair of the fistula or pseudoaneurysm are indicated, as is evacuation of any clot. When done in a timely fashion, outcomes can be gratifying. Later, a secondary operation with nerve action potential

(NAP) recordings may be necessary for plexus element lesions in continuity associated with these vascular lesions, because acute decisions regarding their resection and repair are usually not feasible. Certainly, elements found disrupted or apart in association with vascular injury may merit acute repair but only if the mechanism is sharp by glass or knife. If blunt, repair should be delayed for several weeks so that the extent of resection needed to reach healthy tissue is evident.

Sharp Transection

Another category that merits acute repair (within 72 hours) is sharp transection of a nerve or plexus element. Here, acute repair is certainly indicated. Retraction has had little time to occur, the amount of trimming needed to reach healthy tissue is minimal, and end-to-end suture with minimal tension rather than graft repair is almost always possible. Nerve repair can be done at the same time as repair of injuries to associated structures, such as tendons and vessels.

Blunt Transection

By comparison, a delay of several weeks is indicated for blunt transactions attributable to automobile metal, chain saws, axes, or propeller blades, for example. Here, the force is a blunt one, and there is a variable amount of proximal and distal stump damage. The extent of this injury is unpredictable acutely but becomes evident by 2 to 3 weeks, when inspection of the proximal and

[a] Department of Neurosurgery, Louisiana State University Health Sciences Center, 2020 Gravier Street, New Orleans, LA 70112, USA
[b] Neurosurgery Clinic, Ochsner Hospital, 1514 Jefferson Highway, New Orleans, LA 70121, USA
E-mail address: dkline@lsuhsc.edu

Neurosurg Clin N Am 20 (2009) 24–26
doi:10.1016/j.nec.2008.07.030

distal stumps begins to delineate the extent of resection needed to reach healthy tissue. If the wound is explored acutely, the bluntly transected plexus stumps can be tacked down to adjacent but different fascial planes to maintain length, making it more possible for a delayed end-to-end repair rather than repair by grafts. In these settings, a technically good end-to-end repair with minimal tension always outperforms grafts. Despite the apparent inherent logic in these observations, the author and his colleagues are sent failed acute or primary repairs each year that have seemingly been done well technically but have been done on bluntly transected elements, usually injured by boat propellers, chain saws, or skill saws. At the author's institution, the data for transecting plexus injuries are fairly extensive and strongly support the previously discussed contentions.

INDICATIONS FOR DELAYED REPAIR
Gunshot Wounds

Although penetrating in nature, most gunshot wounds (GSWs) leading to severe neurologic deficit leave the nerve in continuity and injure it by stretch associated with cavitation injury. A few (12%–15%) of these wounds transect one or more nerves or elements; however, because of the nature of the missile tract, they do it in a blunt fashion. Thus, plexus element nerve transaction is seen during acute exploration for vascular, bone, or other soft tissue wounds associated with GSWs, the nerve ends should be tacked to adjacent tissue planes. Subsequent repair is undertaken after a few weeks elapse, just as for other mechanisms of blunt transaction. Roughly one half of civilian GSWs, when gross continuity is maintained, show some definitive evidence of recovery by 3 months after the wound occurs; thus, it makes sense to obtain baseline clinical and electrical examinations (the latter at 2 to 3 weeks to allow for Wallerian degeneration). These examinations should be repeated monthly, and if clinical or electrical recovery does not begin to occur by 2 to 4 months, exploration and intraoperative NAP recordings can be done to determine which elements or nerves need resection and repair and for which ones neurolysis alone should suffice.

The value of such an approach is also illustrated by a relatively large cohort of cases cared for at the Louisiana State University Health Sciences Center (LSUHSC). When recovering NAPs across the lesion were present several months after wounding and outcomes were graded by the LSUHSC scale, neurolysis alone gave a grade 3 or better recovery in more than 90% of cases. By comparison, when no NAP was transmitted, resection and histologic examination of the resected specimen uniformly indicated a neurotmetic lesion, and thus one unlikely to recover spontaneously with further time. Graft repair was more likely in this latter category than end-to-end suture, but the latter was achievable sometimes. Outcomes were as expected for the element involved, age of the lesion, and length of the lesion replaced in the case of grafts.

Stretch/Contusive Injuries: Supraclavicular

By far, this is the largest category of plexus injuries needing or serving as candidates for surgical repair. Management is also the most controversial of all the plexus injuries. Having said this, there are some facts that are often glossed over or forgotten. The first is that somewhat more than 40% of adults presenting with complete or near-complete loss in only the C5 and C6 distribution recover relatively useful function spontaneously. Usually, this is evident or beginning to be evident by 3 to 4 months after the injury and even includes an occasional case in which one root has been avulsed. Early surgery and replacement by grafts or nerve transfers would be premature in this group of patients; yet, there is not a reliable noninvasive method of identifying this subset "out front" or earlier except by careful repetitive clinical and electrodiagnostic follow-up. The circumstances for spontaneous recovery are not as robust for C5, C6, and C7 loss with C8 and T1 sparing, in which the incidence of useful spontaneous recovery decreases to 15% or 16%. Nonetheless, it does occur and sometimes even though one of the three involved roots has studies favoring avulsion. Again, in the author's experience, a 3- to 4-month interval is needed to "winnow out" this group of patients with the potential for spontaneous recovery.

When operated on at 3 to 4 months because of lack of recovery, patients with C5-to-C6 loss or C5-to-C7 loss can have NAP studies and operative somatosensory studies added to operative inspection so that the occasional element with regeneration evident by such a study at this point in time is not falsely resected and repaired. Such an approach permits direct plexus element repair when possible, because operative NAPs, along with section of those elements with flat NAP traces, can differentiate between preganglionic, postganglionic, more lateral rupture or stretch, and regenerative lesions. Such a direct repair, when possible, can then be added to the currently popular nerve transfers to optimize outcomes. In a group of 55 C5-to-C6 stretch injuries operated on in a delayed fashion, 14 patents had neurolysis of one or more plexus elements because of regenerative NAPs. In a group of 75 patients with C5-to-C7 stretch injuries operated on in a delayed fashion, 18 patients had neurolysis of one or more elements because of regenerative NAPs.

Unfortunately, the natural history of flail arm (C5 through T1 loss) is less fortuitous, because only 4% to 5% of patients have spontaneous recovery that is useful. In the author's opinion, this is a group in which earlier surgery is indicated if associated injuries and the overall condition of the patient permit. The incidence of nerve root avulsion in flail arm is higher than in other types of supraclavicular plexus stretch injuries. As a result, the incidence of regenerating NAP recordings is much lower than in other categories of brachial plexus stretch/avulsion injuries. Only a few of the patients in the flail arm group operated on in a delayed fashion had regenerative NAPs. They were usually from C5 or its outflows and less frequently from C6, but there were also occasional exceptions to that trend in other distributions in the 112 patients studied by such recordings. Thus, the need for nerve transfer or intraplexal neurotization is higher in flail arm than in other groups of stretch injuries. Nonetheless, in only 5% of patients are all roots avulsed, and in many patients, C5 is usable for direct repair after operative recordings exclude preganglionic or regenerative activity. In some cases, C6 is also available for direct repair to add to any nerve transfer to be done. Of course, the need for NAP recordings is less in the flail arm group than in those with C5-to-C6 or C5-to-C7 patterns of loss; however, when NAP recordings are used, they work best after a few months rather than more acutely. Outcomes in these supraclavicular stretch/avulsion injuries are available, at least from the approach used by the author and his colleagues, and some attempt to use the previously discussed timing guidelines. The major problem is delay in referral, and that needs to be corrected somehow for this large group of patients.

Infraclavicular Stretch/Contusive Injuries

Some of these injuries undergo spontaneous improvement. Infraclavicular plexus injuries are associated with a high incidence of associated injuries to major vessels, bones, and other soft tissues. Occasionally, these associated injuries require an acute operation and correction. If infraclavicular element(s) are pulled apart (which is usually not the case), delayed repair is once again indicated, as it is for those in continuity. Visual inspection alone cannot reliably differentiate a nonconducting neuroma-in-continuity requiring repair from a recovering neuroma-in-continuity requiring only external neurolysis. These observations necessitate a delay before exploration for the infraclavicular plexus stretch/compression or GSW injury so as to allow recovering axons to regrow across the lesion. This concept is supported in the author and his colleagues' series of axillary nerve injuries, in which 17 of 86 patients with complete clinical and electromyographic (EMG) loss 5 or more months after the injury had an NAP transmitted across their lesion in continuity and had neurolysis alone (n = 15) or split repair (n = 2), with an averaged outcome LSUHSC grade of 4.0. Distribution of findings and results was equally good for lateral and posterior cord injuries and their outflows but was, of course, poorer for medial cord and medial cord–to–ulnar nerve injuries. Had all these recovering neuromas been excised soon after injury and subjected to graft repair without delayed NAP evaluation, the results would have been substantially worse.

Iatrogenic Injuries

Management of these injuries follows the same principles as for other types of peripheral nerve injuries. For example, elements transected by a scalpel or scissors are ideally treated with acute repair. Blunt transaction attributable to Bovie or other instrumentation is repaired after a few weeks have elapsed. Injuries attributable to retraction/compression/stretch are likely to result in lesions in continuity and are explored if possible after a 3- to 4-month delay. This strategy permits operative NAP recordings to guide the need for graft repair versus external neurolysis. Regrettably, referral of iatrogenic nerve injuries typically are needlessly delayed for a prolonged period in the hope that spontaneous recovery might obviate the need for another operation.

Nerve Transfers for Severe Nerve Injury

Bassam M.J. Addas, MBChB, FRCSC[a], Rajiv Midha, MD, MSc, FRSCS[b],*

KEYWORDS

- Accessory nerve • Brachial plexus injury
- Intercostal nerves • Neurotization • Spinal nerve

Brachial plexus and other severe nerve injuries can have devastating consequences affecting largely a young, productive population. The optimal management, whenever possible, is direct nerve repair, which can be difficult or impossible to achieve in patients who have spinal nerve root avulsion or very proximal injury, and in patients who have a large nerve gap. Delay in presentation for surgery further complicates the situation. Nerve transfer is one strategy with potential for improved outcome. Nerve transfers (also referred to as "neurotization" or "nerve crossing") involve the repair of a distal denervated nerve element using a proximal foreign nerve as the donor of neurons and their axons, which will reinnervate the distal targets. The concept is to sacrifice the function of a lesser-valued donor muscle to revive function in the recipient nerve and muscle that will undergo reinnervation.[1] The first report of neurotization in an attempt to restore injured plexus function was by Tuttle[2] in 1913. Popularized by Oberlin, distal fascicular nerve transfers are showing encouraging and promising results,[3] and are gradually replacing the tediously performed proximal brachial plexus exploration and lengthy graft repair, which have more unpredictable results.

NERVE TRANSFERS: INDICATIONS, PROS, AND CONS

Currently, no absolute guidelines exist for when nerve transfer should be performed, but the authors consider the following to be appropriate conditions in which nerve transfer can be useful:

- Brachial plexus roots avulsion or very proximal intraforaminal injury close to the spinal cord with no, or poor, nerve stump available to lead nerve graft from
- Proximal injury with a long distance to the target muscle (eg, a high [axillary or arm] ulnar nerve lesion)
- Significant vascular and or bony injuries in the region of the brachial plexus; keeping away from of the injured, scarred area may avoid unnecessary damage to vital structures
- Delayed presentation and long interval from injury to surgery; the ideal time for direct nerve repair is up to 6 months after the injury
- Previously failed brachial plexus or proximal nerve repair

The following are some useful criteria for choosing donor nerves for transfer:

- Donor nerve near motor end plate of the target muscle
- Expandable or redundant donor nerve
- Donor nerve with many pure motor (or sensory) axons
- Donor nerve with synergistic action to the target muscle, when possible, to facilitate motor reeducation
- Size matching between the donor and recipient nerves

[a] Division of Neurosurgery, Department of Surgery, King Abdulaziz University Hospital, P.O. Box 80215, Jeddah 21589, Kingdom of Saudi Arabia
[b] Division of Neurosurgery, Department of Clinical Neurosciences, Room 1195, 1403 29th Street NW, Foothills Medical Centre, University of Calgary, Calgary, AB T2L 2T9, Canada
* Corresponding author.
E-mail address: rajmidha@ucalgary.ca (R. Midha).

Neurosurg Clin N Am 20 (2009) 27–38
doi:10.1016/j.nec.2008.07.018

The advantages of using a nerve transfer over a nerve graft repair include the following:

Nerve transfers are usually done with the donor nerve brought closer to the end-organ. The closer the innervation of the target muscle, the shorter the distance the regenerating axons have to travel and subsequently, the better the chance of functional reinnervation. It allows improved and earlier reinnervation with potentially improved outcomes.

Most nerve transfers can be accomplished without the use of an interposition graft. This advantage translates into one microsuture repair site, compared with two, and a correspondingly decreased likelihood of loss of axons (or their misdirection) at the repair sites

When selection is made carefully and functional recovery takes place, nerve transfer seems an ideal option with few downsides. However, it is not a flawless technique. Some of the disadvantages include

Donor site morbidity and loss of muscle function of the donor nerve, particularly so when the donor nerve or fascicle is sacrificed to a muscle with suboptimal function to begin with. For instance, taking an ulnar nerve fascicle in a patient who has poor (grade 3 or barely grade 4) hand function may significantly downgrade finger flexion and intrinsic hand muscles.

The muscle whose nerve has been used for transfer will be no longer suitable for muscle transfer. Examples are the latissmus dorsi (thoracodorsal nerve [TDN]), pectoralis major (medial pectoral nerve), and the triceps muscles (triceps muscle branch), all of which can be used to restore elbow flexion.

The need for central reeducation to have functional recovery[4–6]

Nerve transfers tend to take the surgeon away from exploring the injury site, the brachial plexus, which carries the potential for surgeons to not even offer an anatomic nerve reconstruction, even in situations when these are perfectly appropriate. An example is to perform a distal triceps fascicle to axillary nerve transfer in a patient who a posterior cord–axillary nerve stretch lesion, which fares well with resection of the intervening neuroma and nerve graft repair.[7]

With the increasing use of transfers, newly trained peripheral nerve surgeons are less likely to have exposure to the brachial plexus and they will be increasingly unfamiliar with the detailed anatomy and intraoperative electrophysiology assessment of the lesions.

TREATMENT OPTIONS FOR BRACHIAL PLEXUS INJURIES

Generally, the main objectives in treating severe brachial plexus injury are to restore shoulder abduction, external rotation, elbow flexion, and forearm supination.[8] The combination of these movements will allow the patient to hold a food tray, to bring his/her hand up to his/her mouth, and to be able to push doors open while carrying items with the healthy arm. Some experts also advocate attempting restoration of wrist extension and shoulder adduction.[9,10] The following are some of the authors' preferred options for nerve reconstruction.

C5-C6 (Upper Trunk) Palsy

Traumatic complete avulsion of C5 is uncommon; therefore, C5 can often be used for plexoplexal repairs with interposed sural nerve grafts.[8] The information from preoperative imaging (CT post myelogram or high-quality MRI scans), supplemented with intraoperative dissection to the level of the intervertebral foramen and the use of intraoperative electrodiagnostic studies, will aid in the decision making.[11–14] Nonetheless, nerve transfer may be preferred because of its quicker recovery and avoidance of the injury site dissection, which can be tedious and fruitless.[9,15] Distal spinal accessory nerve (SAN) transfer to the suprascapular nerve (**Fig. 1**) and triceps branch transfer to the anterior division of the axillary nerve will restore shoulder abduction.[16,17] Elbow flexion is restored by transferring an ulnar nerve fascicle (selecting a fascicle that predominantly supplies flexor carpi ulnaris muscle) to biceps branch ± a median nerve fascicle to the brachialis branch of the musculocutaneous nerve.[3,18]

C5, C6, and C7 Palsy

When C7 is involved and the triceps muscle is weak (Medical Research Council [MRC] grade<4), triceps branch-axillary nerve transfer may downgrade the triceps muscle further and therefore, should not be used. The same overall strategy used in C5 and C6 injury can be used. However, to reinnervate the axillary nerve, thoracodorsal nerve (TDN), if intact, can be used. Medial pectoral nerve and intercostal nerves (ICNs) are alternative donors. Furthermore, the triceps muscle, if significantly weak, can be reanimated by transferring ICNs to the triceps fascicle of the radial nerve or directly to the triceps muscle branches (whichever is weaker).[15]

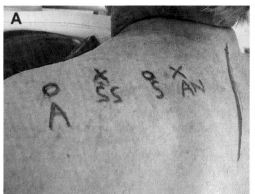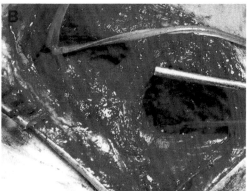

Fig.1. (A) A patient is seen positioned prone with a left superior scapular incision outlined. This positioning allows exposure of both the accessory nerve (AN), which is located midway between the spinous process of the vertebra (vertical line is the midline) and the medial spine of the scapula (S), and the suprascapular (SS) nerve, landmarked halfway between the acromion (A) and the medial spine of the scapula (S). (B) The distal accessory nerve deep to the trapezius muscle (encircled by two vessel loops) and, to the right, the suprascapular nerve deep and just proximal to the suprascapular notch after incising the transverse scapular ligament.

Total Plexus (C5-T1) Palsy

Although a pan-plexus injury is the most common situation, avulsion of all C5-T1 roots is rare; the C5 spinal nerve root may be singularly spared, thus allowing it to be used as the source of axons for a plexo-plexal repair to distal elements.[8] Overall, in this dreadful situation, the donor nerve options are limited to extraplexal nerves. Donor nerves include the spinal accessory, phrenic, ICNs, contralateral C7, and the disparately anterior motor divisions of the cervical plexus.[8] The reanimation of hand function is disappointingly poor and no attempt is made to reinnervate the lower plexus elements in adults. Secondary reconstructive procedures are usually needed for functional recovery of the hand.

In this difficult scenario, the author's strategy will depend on the availability of the C5 nerve root. If intact, C5 to upper trunk elements (suprascapular and to axillary nerve) is performed using sural nerve grafts. At times, C5 (if robust) may also be directed by way of a graft to the musculocutaneous nerve. However, elbow flexion is usually restored by performing intercostal-musculocutaneous (ICN-MC) nerve transfers (**Fig. 2**).[19] When C5 is not available for use, accessory-suprascapular nerve transfer is used as means of restoring some useful shoulder abduction, together with ICN-MC nerve transfer.

In addition to the criteria listed earlier for choosing the donor nerve for transfer, personal surgical preference and the experience of the different institutes are believed to play a role in this choice. Examples are the C7 and phrenic nerve transfer, with most of the reports coming from China and

Taiwan[20–25] with good results; such reports are rarely reported by North American centers.

COMMON NERVES USED FOR NERVE TRANSFERS
Spinal Accessory Nerve

As an extraplexal nerve, the SAN is rarely injured in patients who have brachial plexus injury. When harvested distal to its initial trapezius motor branches

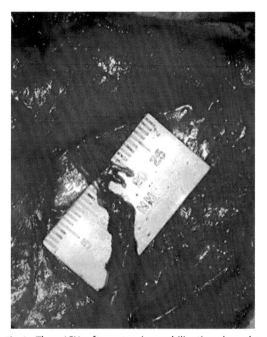

Fig. 2. Three ICNs after extensive mobilization along the chest wall, tunneled behind the right axillary skin fold and ready to be coapted directly (without interposed nerve grafts) to the musculocutaneous nerve.

and transferred to the donor nerves, it provides a good source of motor axons (1500–3000 myelinated axons) to the plexal elements, with and without the use of an interposition graft.[15] The SAN is commonly transferred to suprascapular and musculocutaneous nerves to restore shoulder abduction and elbow flexion, respectively. For restoration of dynamic shoulder function, the suprascapular and axillary nerves have been chosen as targets. Although the former can be repaired directly by end-end suture of the distal accessory nerve, the latter requires an interposed nerve graft.[26]

SAN transfer to the suprascapular nerve to restore shoulder abduction has been associated with mixed results; some investigators reported good functional recovery when SAN was transferred to the suprascapular nerve alone or when combined with axillary nerve reinnervation.[27] Malessy and associates[28] had more pessimistic results, with poor restoration of active glenohumeral abduction; their patients compensate by rotating the scapula laterally (thoracoscapular rotation) to achieve and maintain their shoulder abduction. Suprascapular nerve reanimation alone may restore up to a mean range of 90° of shoulder abduction, and such range of motion has been claimed to be useful by some;[27] however, when combined with axillary nerve reanimation, a more functional recovery, with up to 115°,[17] can be restored.

The other major target for accessory nerve transfer has been the musculocutaneous nerve. The results for elbow flexion in recent series have been good, with MRC grade 3 or better outcomes achieved in 65%,[29] 72%,[30] 72.5%,[31] and 83%[32] of patients. In the analysis of factors predicting outcome, the most important negative predictor was increased duration of time between injury and surgery; the need for a longer graft also negatively influenced results.[9,11] Although a meta-analysis of the literature suggests that when the musculocutaneous nerve is the recipient nerve, it is best to use ICNs as donors,[33] only the series by Waikakul and colleagues[32] directly compared the two extraplexal donors, finding that the accessory nerve achieved superior outcomes for elbow flexion compared with the ICNs.[11]

Traditionally, accessory to suprascapular nerve transfer has been accomplished through an anterior supraclavicular approach; however, more recently, a posterior approach (see **Fig. 1**) has been described, particularly when triceps branch to axillary nerve transfer is considered in combination.[34]

Intercostal Nerves

ICNs are commonly used extraplexal donor nerves. They have a long history of use and have been successfully transferred to the musculocutaneous nerve with satisfactory results.[19] The importance of this transfer becomes especially evident in patients who have severe brachial plexus injury involving C5-T1 roots, where the source of donor nerves is limited. ICNs are mixed motor/sensory nerves, with 500 to 700 myelinated motor axons. When an average of three nerves is used, an adequate number of motor axons will be available for transfer.

Results of ICN-MC nerve transfer vary widely with the various techniques, ranging from no change in biceps function to strong elbow flexion. The differences in the techniques involve

Site of ICN transection ranging from paravertebral to parasternal
Number of ICNs used
The recipient nerve
Use of interposition graft
Use of vascularized ICN

Given that few patients are reported and the various permutations used in these techniques, it is difficult to agree on the optimum transfer technique.

Standardized techniques, consisting of the use of three ICNs (third to fifth) to the distal musculocutaneous nerve, without interposed grafts, used by Friedman and colleagues[35] and the Duke University group, led to more consistent results, approaching MRC grade 3 or better function in about 50% of the patients. Their research also provided the first detailed evidence of independent (without synkinetic respiratory movements) use of biceps over the course of time, hinting at cortical plasticity, a concept that has subsequently been directly validated with electrophysiologic and functional brain mapping and imaging studies.[4–6,36] Indeed, it is suggested that whether patients obtain functional use depends on cortical readaptation, with failures construed to lack such adaptation; however, this hypothesis requires validation.[15] In a recent meta-analysis, ICN-MC transfer resulted in 72% of patients recovering to greater than or equal to M3 strength, but only 47% of patients recovering to that strength when an interposition graft was used. Restoration of elbow flexion was superior when compared with accessory-musculocutaneous transfer.[12] In a small group comparison, Okinaga and Nagano[37] did not find any clinical advantage to using vascularized versus nonvascularized ICN transfer.

Unilateral (ICN) transfer does not significantly impair respiratory function. However, most peripheral nerve surgeons generally agree that respiratory dysfunction will occur when the phrenic nerve is simultaneously transferred. This old belief is currently being challenged repeatedly.[38]

Ipsilateral and Contralateral C7 Spinal Nerve Transfer

The C7 spinal nerve, middle trunk, and its anterior and posterior divisions can be used as a donor nerves in cases of partial or complete brachial plexus injury. Ipsilateral and contralateral sides can be used according to the pattern of injury. The C7 nerve root provides a rich source of nerve fibers because it contains up to 23,000 axons. C7 contains between four and six fascicles, continues as the middle trunk, and subsequently divides into anterior and posterior divisions. The anterior division contains laterally disposed fascicles with more motor supply (especially to pectoralis) and medial fascicles with more sensory axons, whereas the posterior division contains motor input for the extensor muscles (mainly triceps). Such an orientation allows a better selection when choosing the recipient nerves. The whole root, or part of it, can be used with minimal or no deficit in the donor side.[21]

In some cases of Erb's palsy, where both C5 and C6 are avulsed, the C7 spinal nerve is intact and available as an intraplexal donor for reinnervating the distal upper trunk or its divisional outflow. Such a transfer can be associated with good outcomes related to the recipient elements,[39] with little risk for loss of function from taking the C7 spinal nerve.[22] However, considerable caution is required if significant lower plexus lesion coexists because the muscles innervated by C7, which normally would be redundantly supplied by the C8 (and T1) spinal nerves, will not be present.

The redundancy of the C7 spinal nerve, allowing for its safe sacrifice, has been verified by investigators who have used the contralateral C7 as a donor for transfer. Other than causing mild loss of triceps function and clinically inconsequential loss of the triceps reflex, the procedure appears to be safe as far as motor loss is concerned. However, sensory abnormalities are common following C7 sacrifice, and may be permanent in 5% of cases.[40] Moreover, neuropathic pain may be evoked temporarily in a few patients,[41] and a rare case may have permanent motor deficits in wrist extension.[42] Selective use of anterior or posterior portions of the contralateral C7, aided by intraoperative electrophysiologic tests, may make the procedure safer and further add to the specificity of the reinnervated element to which it is transferred.[21,23]

The best results in the use of contralateral C7 for total avulsion were claimed by Waikakul and colleagues[32] who noted that, in 98 adolescent and adult patients, when the median nerve was the recipient, good sensory function was achieved in about half of the adolescents and some also experienced forearm muscle recovery. In a most carefully reported 3-year follow-up, Songchareon and colleagues[26] reported median nerve motor recovery to an MRC grade 3 or 4 in about 20% of patients, whereas another 20% had an MRC grade 2 outcome in wrist flexion. Outcome in the sensory domain was better, especially in adolescents, with half of these patients having useful sensory restoration in the median nerve distribution. In Terzis and colleagues'[39] adult brachial plexus series, the average grade achieved in various recipients was less than MRC 3. Others have used the C7 strictly to transfer, by way of vascularized ulnar nerve graft, to the lateral cord contribution to the median nerve and report a 100% success rate with good sensory recovery.

Contralateral C7 nerve transfer has been used recently in 12 infants and children, with promising results.[43] A more selective approach of choosing the motor rootlets through a posterior approach has recently been described, with promising results.[10,39]

One of the main criticisms of this transfer technique remains the long graft (and hence regeneration) distance, but the possibility of a prespinal retropharyngeal route of graft placement has been suggested.[44] Nevertheless, the technique remains limited, given the modest results in motor recovery. The synchronous movement of the healthy side required to facilitate the desired action can be frustrating, with patients needing to make a fist on the healthy side to initiate the action on the involved side. This facilitatory action may take up to 3 years to improve but rarely will it go away completely.[28] Although most of the reports suggest minimal or no deficit in the donor side, even a minor deficit in the only normal arm can be of considerable clinical and psychologic consequence. Perhaps a targeted approach to obtain median nerve distribution sensory recovery is warranted, although similar outcomes may be possible with a less cumbersome transfer from the lower ICNs to the sensory (lateral cord) contribution to the median nerve.[45] The authors, therefore, rarely, if ever, perform contralateral C7 transfers.

Medial Pectoral Nerves

The pectoralis major muscle has dual input from the medial and lateral pectoral nerves, arising from the medial and lateral cords, respectively.

Because C5 and C6 avulsion interrupts the lateral cord supply, the muscle remains innervated (and strong) as long as a significant injury to the C7 and C8 elements does not occur. Although popularized recently for upper plexus injuries, the medial pectoral nerve as a donor for transfer has been considered previously and used infrequently, as reviewed by Narakas[46] for adults and Gilbert[47] for obstetric palsy.

Brandt and Mackinnon[48] directed the medial pectoral nerve to the musculocutaneous nerve, with the additional innovation of turning the distal lateral antebrachial cutaneous nerve (the cutaneous derivative of the musculocutaneous) into the biceps muscle to try to avoid loss of motor axons into the cutaneous distribution. A resurgence of interest in this transfer has been associated with reports of useful outcomes (defined as MRC grade 3 or better) in elbow flexion in approximately 84% of patients.[49] Excellent results in obstetric palsy, too, have been claimed, with success in 68% of cases.[50] However, the results of various series vary, and Samardzic and associates[29] have noted that medial pectoral transfers were associated with significantly improved outcomes in elbow flexion as compared with ICN and accessory nerve transfers. This group has also been one of the few to demonstrate remarkably good results in transfer to the axillary nerve, reporting useful results in more than 80% of patients.[49]

With the increasing interest in the medial pectoral nerve as a donor, the anatomy of the pectoral nerve complex has been more clearly defined.[51] The traditional concept of separate lateral and medial pectoral nerves innervating the pectoralis minor and major muscles as discrete nerves has been replaced with the knowledge that as these nerves run toward the pectoralis minor and major muscles, they exhibit considerable branching and intermingling. Not infrequently, a plexus will form where branches from the medial and lateral pectoral nerves, destined for the pectoralis major, merge together and then final branches will ramify toward the muscle. Because only one, or at times two, of these terminal branches to the pectoralis need be taken (and distally) for the transfer, the practical implication is that some pectoralis major supply can be preserved and a direct repair without intervening graft can be performed to the musculocutaneous nerve in the distal axilla. Significant caution needs to be exercised if substantial injury involving C7 and C8 exists; in this case, pectoralis major will be weak preoperatively and this finding is a contraindication to considering a medial pectoral transfer. A similar sophisticated appreciation of the nerve supply of the biceps and brachialis muscles[52] has propelled further surgical evolution

in transfers so that the biceps and brachialis are discretely reinnervated by transfer procedures.[18]

Phrenic Nerve

The phrenic nerve is the motor nerve to the diaphragm, originating mainly from the fourth cervical root, but both C3 and C5 contribute to and augment the nerve. For a complete phrenic nerve paralysis to take place, both C4 and C5 have to be injured. This scenario is, fortunately, not common because the C4, like C5, nerve root is strongly bound with fibrous tissue to the chute-like structure of the transverse process. In 100 consecutive cases of brachial plexus injury, Chen and others[53] have found an incidence of 13% severely and 7% partially injured phrenic nerves. When healthy, unlike the cervical plexus, which contains a variable and small aliquot of motor fibers, the phrenic nerve contains many pure motor axons that allow the possibility of entire or partial transfer with success.

Box 1 compares the advantages and disadvantages of using the phrenic nerve as a donor for transfers. In 12 patients, a 75% success rate with phrenic transfer to musculocutaneous, suprascapular, or axillary nerves was reported.[54] In particular, the transfer to the musculocutaneous nerve has been an excellent tactic, with 11/12 patients achieving better than antigravity (MRC

Box 1
Advantages and disadvantages of phrenic nerve transfer

Advantages

Predominance of motor axons

Proximity to major nerves, namely the suprascapular and musculocutaneous nerves, which may allow a direct coaptation, sometimes, with no intervening graft

Technical ease of finding and dissecting

Disadvantages

The potential for significant respiratory function decline, at least temporarily, and the poor handling of respiratory infections, particularly in the pediatric age group or in adults with poor cardiorespiratory functions

The short length of nerve available from the usual supraclavicular approach, with a graft usually needed

The need for considerable neural plasticity because the patient will need to take a deep breath when he/she tries to flex his/her elbow; although this situation may improve over 2 to 3 years, it can be a frustrating task for patients

grade 3) and 58% MRC grade 4 function.[55] An important issue when the phrenic nerve is sacrificed is the resulting respiratory function compromise, which has been measured to be an average of about a 10% decrease in vital capacity.[55] Although not clinically important in most situations, this degree of loss in respiratory reserve will produce symptoms in higher-demand situations and may be severely detrimental to infants and children who develop respiratory infections. This possibility essentially precludes the use of the phrenic nerve as a donor in infants who are undergoing nerve reconstruction for obstetric palsy. Moreover, it also implies that the ICNs should not be used as donors for transfer when the phrenic nerve function is absent preoperatively or when the phrenic is transferred.

Xu and associates[23] compared vascularized and nonvascularized phrenic nerve transfer in 15 patients and found no statistically significant difference. This lack of difference was attributed to the small diameter of the nerve (2 mm) and its well-vascularized bed. It is not completely understood, but Luedemann and collaborators[55] found a statistically significant drop in vital capacity when using the right phrenic nerve compared with the left. This difference was not clinically significant, but the investigators cautioned against using the right side if the maximal inspiratory pressure is decreased preoperatively. It was not clear why patients who have phrenic nerve transfer fare well regarding the respiratory function, but it has been attributed in part to the presence of accessory phrenic nerve. However, Xu and colleagues[25] showed that patients will recover vital capacity within 1 year following section of the phrenic nerve near its attachment to the diaphragm done thoracosopically, a technique that

rules out the role of accessory phrenic nerve supply. Transferring both phrenic and ICNs is not preferred because the patient is deprived of two important nerves that supply the diaphragm and the accessory respiratory muscles, respectively. This principle has been challenged recently in 15 patients who had both nerves transferred; some also had the spinal accessory and cervical plexus motor branches used as donors, thus denervating many accessory respiratory muscles. Although the patients' diaphragmatic and lung function showed a measurable impact, their ventilation and exercise performance were not affected.[38]

Ulnar Nerve Fascicle Transfer (Oberlin Transfer)

In 1994, Oberlin and associates[3] reported the use of an ulnar nerve fascicle for transfer to the biceps muscle branch. Since Oberlin's first description of this technique, transferring an ulnar nerve fascicle has become a commonly used nerve transfer for biceps muscle reanimation. The ulnar nerve receives its input from C8 and T1, with occasional contribution from C7. These roots are usually preserved in patients who have upper plexus injury. The ulnar nerve is anatomically close to the biceps muscle and its branch; this anatomic fact allows a direct coaptation of the two nerves (**Fig. 3**). The nerve is exposed in the medial arm and commonly found in a groove between the biceps and triceps muscles. Once identified and isolated using a nerve stimulator, the common epineurium of the ulnar nerve is opened under magnification, and the fascicle, with predominant innervation to the flexor carpi ulnaris muscle, is isolated and used for transfer to the biceps branch. Intraoperative stimulation using a disposable variable

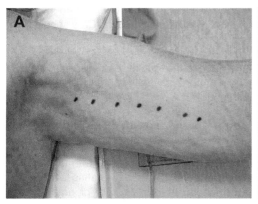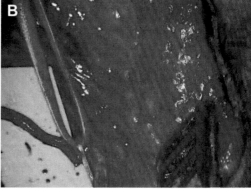

Fig. 3. (A) The incision (dotted line) at the medial arm between biceps and triceps muscles for the exposure of ulnar and musculocutaneous nerves. (B) An ulnar nerve fascicle (electrically verified as predominantly supplying flexor carpi ulnaris muscle) isolated (vessel loop) and ready to be coapted to the biceps branch (overlying the blue background) of musculocutaneous nerve.

stimulating device (Xomed, Medtronics Corporation) is usually sufficient for the identification of an appropriate fascicle.

Leechavengvongs and colleagues[56] reported 32 patients with mean time to surgery of 6 months and follow-up of 18 months, with 93% of patients recovering elbow flexion to MRC grade 4, and no patient showing ulnar nerve–associated hand function deterioration.

More impressive results have been those reported by Sungpet,[57] who used a single ulnar nerve fascicle directed to biceps and obtained an MRC grade 3 or better outcome in 34/36 patients. Noted, too, in his article, was that time to reinnervation began as early as 3.3 months and that hand function and ulnar assessment using a series of tests and functional tools was not compromised in long-term follow-up. The key aspect of the procedure is to reinnervate the biceps branch close to its motor entry into the muscle.

A recent report indicates that elbow flexion function will be further augmented (especially in delayed surgery cases) by concomitantly reinnervating the brachialis muscle by way of a graft from the medial pectoral nerve.[58] A similar promising result has been reported in obstetric brachial plexus palsy.

Partial Median Nerve Fascicle Transfer

The same concept of transferring a fascicle from the ulnar nerve can be applied to the median nerve by choosing a fascicle innervating predominantly flexor carpi radialis or palmaris longus muscles. The median nerve receives contributions from upper and lower plexus elements and therefore can be partially involved in patients who have upper plexus palsies; however, it may not always be suitable for fascicle transfer because it may produce more deficits in the distribution of the median nerve. Sungpet and colleagues[59] reported using a single median nerve fascicle, which predominantly innervated either the flexor carpi radialis or palmaris longus muscle, and transferring it to the biceps motor branch of the musculocutaneous nerve. They observed MRC grade 4 elbow flexion in four out of five patients and MRC grade 3 recovery in one patient. No donor nerve morbidity occurred. In a report by Ferraresi and associates,[60] elbow flexion was restored by using median nerve fascicle to main musculocutaneous nerve in only 4 of 43 patients, so the authors caution against a nondiscrete transfer. Mackinnon[61] used median nerve fascicle to brachialis branch and ulnar nerve fascicle to biceps branch (so-called "double fascicular transfer") to augment elbow flexion. The investigator's rationale was explained by the fact that brachialis is the main elbow flexor and biceps is primarily a supinator with flexion being a secondary function, thus making reanimating the brachialis an important component of reconstruction of elbow flexion. The authors' preferred technique is to use the Oberlin transfer alone in most cases, but to consider a double fascicular transfer in delayed (>6 months postinjury) cases. They also caution against using these transfers in cases where the patient's preoperative ulnar or median nerve is compromised.

Triceps Muscle Branch to Axillary Nerve

The triceps muscle, with its three heads, offers the possibility of using one of the three nerve branches as a good donor nerve to the nearby axillary nerve. When the triceps is of normal power, the nerve supply of one of its heads can be transferred without any demonstrable loss in its strength. Leechavengvongs and associates[17] described transferring the long head of the triceps branch to the anterior division of the axillary nerve (**Fig. 4**) in seven patients, combined with accessory-suprascapular nerves, with excellent outcome in shoulder abduction. Colbert and Mackinnon[34] have recently reported a posterior approach, in which both transfers were performed in a prone position (see **Fig. 1**).

Although no firm agreement exists as to the importance of each of the triceps heads, it seems that muscle weakness is a rare occurrence, regardless of the chosen branch, providing the muscle is of normal power. The branch to the medial head is easy to find between the lateral and the long heads, and has enough length for coaptation to the axillary nerve. The branch to the long head of the triceps is closer to the axillary nerve, but division of the teres major muscle is almost always required to obtain adequate length.[47] The author's choice of the anterior division of the axillary nerve versus the axillary nerve proper depends on each patient's individual anatomy. Care should be exercised not to use this technique in patients who have triceps weakness or C7 injury because it may affect the quality of the donor nerve and, most importantly, will worsen the triceps muscle strength.

Distal Anterior Interosseous Branch Transfer-Deep Motor Branch of Ulnar Nerve

Proximal ulnar nerve injuries with loss of intrinsic hand muscles are a devastating event with severe functional loss. Primary or grafted repair of high ulnar nerve injury is typically associated with inadequate or no recovery of hand intrinsic muscle function.[62] In high ulnar nerve injury, the long distance between the cell body and the

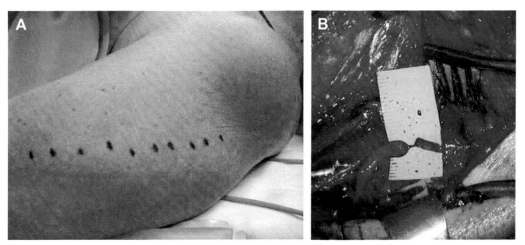

Fig. 4. (*A*) A posterior arm incision marked between the atrophic deltoid muscle and the long head of triceps allows for simultaneous exposure of both triceps branches of the radial nerve and distal axillary nerve. (*B*) Anterior division of the axillary nerve is ready to be coapted to the long head of triceps branch. Note the slight difference in diameter of the two nerve stumps.

target muscle prevents a timely reinnervation of target muscles. Nerve transfer presents a good treatment option for high ulnar nerve injury because it avoids the long distance the regenerating axons have to travel. The pronator quadratus muscle branch (of the distal anterior interosseous nerve) offers a suitable donor nerve for the deep motor branch of the ulnar nerve because it is purely motor (900 axons), is close to the deep motor branch of the ulnar nerve (1200 axons), and is a good size match (**Fig. 5**). Loss of pronator quadratus muscle is usually not clinically noticeable.[63] Novak and Mackinnon[63] reported eight patients who had ulnar

nerve injury proximal to the elbow; all patients demonstrated reinnervation of ulnar intrinsic hand muscles, with improved lateral pinch and grip strength. No functional deficit in pronation was reported. Battiston and Lanzetta[62] reported seven patients who had double median to ulnar nerve transfer in which the distal anterior interosseous branch was transferred to the deep motor branch of the ulnar nerve and the palmar cutaneous branch of the median nerve was transferred to the sensory branch of the ulnar nerve. Six of the seven patients recovered to grade M4 or better. All patients recovered protective sensation, and five had full sensory recovery.

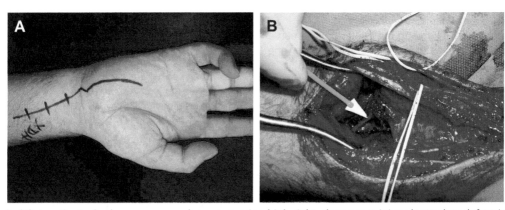

Fig. 5. (*A*) A patient who has a severe and nonrecovering high right ulnar nerve injury (note claw deformity of little finger) is prepared for an incision to expose the deep motor branch of the ulnar nerve and distal anterior interosseous nerve. (*B*) The motor branch of the ulnar nerve is extensively neurolyzed (topmost vessel loops) so that it can be sectioned proximally. It will then be brought in approximation to the deeply located distal anterior interosseous nerve branch to the pronator quadratus muscle (*arrow*).

Thoracodorsal Nerve

The TDN is a pure motor nerve supplying the latissmus dorsi muscle; it receives input from C6 to C8. The mean surgical available length for transfer is 12.3 cm with a range of 8.5 to 19 cm, with diameter ranges from 2.1 to 3 mm. The number of myelinated axons ranges from 1530 to 2470. All these criteria make the nerve an excellent motor nerve donor. Transfer of the TDN to the musculocutaneous and to the axillary nerves has been achieved successfully.[64,65] The available length of the TDN allows its coaptation to those nerves without the need of an interposition graft. However, in patients who have C7, middle trunk, or posterior cord injury, the TDN may be significantly affected. Clinical examination of the latissmus dorsi muscle, electromyographic testing, and intraoperative stimulation will allow an accurate assessment before selecting TDN as a donor nerve. Using TDN will lead to latissmus dorsi muscle weakness and subsequently, arm adduction, an action that can be helpful in children age group as they use it to hold objects under their armpits. Notably, it also takes away the option of using this muscle for transfer to augment elbow flexion.

Use of Nerve Transfer for Restoration of Sensation

Nerve transfer to restore sensation is much less commonly used than motor nerve transfer. However, the same principles apply. The sensory nerve transfer can be a useful procedure when restoring protective sensation is the goal.[66] Examples of sensory nerve transfer include

Palmar cutaneous branch of the median nerve to the ulnar nerve sensory branch

Deep peroneal nerve at the ankle level to the medial plantar nerve

Saphenous nerve to the posterior tibial nerve

Digital nerves of the little (radial side) or ring fingers to the thumb or index fingers

Intercostal (sensory) nerves to the lateral cord (which is primarily sensory) head to the median nerve

REFERENCES

1. Narakas A, Hentz VR. Neurotization in brachial plexus injuries. Indication and results. Clin Orthop 1988;237:43–56.
2. Tuttle HK. Exposure of the brachial plexus with nerve transplantation. JAMA 1913;61:15–7.
3. Oberlin C, Beal D, Leechavengvongs S, et al. Nerve transfer to biceps muscle using a part of ulnar nerve for C5-C6 avulsion of the brachial plexus: anatomical study and report of four cases. J Hand Surg [Am] 1994;19(2):232–7.
4. Malessy M, Bakker D, Dekker A. Functional magnetic resonance imaging and control over the biceps muscle after intercostal-musculocutaneous nerve transfer. J Neurosurg 2003;98:261–8.
5. Malessy M, Thomeer R, van Dijk J. Changing central nervous system control following intercostal nerve transfer. J Neurosurg 1998;89:568–74.
6. Malessy M, van der Kamp W, Thomeer R. Cortical excitability of the biceps muscle after intercostal-to-musculocutaneous nerve transfers. Neurosurgery 1998;42:787–95.
7. Kline DG, Kim DH. Axillary nerve repair in 99 patients with 101 stretch injuries. J Neurosurg 2003; 99(4):630–6.
8. Midha R. Nerve transfers for severe brachial plexus injuries: a review. Neurosurg Focus 2004;16(5):E5.
9. Weber R, Mackinnon S. Nerve transfers in the upper extremity. Journal of the American Society for Surgery of the Hand 2004;4(3):200–13.
10. Bertelli JA, Ghizoni MF. Contralateral motor rootlets and ipsilateral nerve transfers in brachial plexus reconstruction. J Neurosurg 2004;101(5):770–8.
11. Kim DH, Cho YJ, Tiel RL, et al. Outcomes of surgery in 1019 brachial plexus lesions treated at Louisiana State University Health Sciences Center. J Neurosurg 2003;98(5):1005–16.
12. Waikakul S, Orapin S, Vanadurongwan V. Clinical results of contralateral C7 root neurotization to the median nerve in brachial plexus injuries with total root avulsions. J Hand Surg [Br] 1999;16(24):556–60.
13. Kline DG, Hackett ER, May P. Evaluation of nerve injuries by evoked potentials and electromyography. J Neurosurg 1969;31:128–36.
14. Kline DG, Hackett ER. Management of the neuroma in continuity. In: Wilkins RH, Rengachary SS, editors. Neurosurgery. New York: McGraw Hill; 1984. p. 1864–71.
15. Wood M, Murray P. Heterotopic nerve transfers: recent trends with expanding indication. J Hand Surg [Am] 2007;32(3):397–408.
16. Bertelli JA, Ghizoni MF. Reconstruction of C5 and C6 brachial plexus avulsion injury by multiple nerve transfers: spinal accessory to suprascapular, ulnar fascicles to biceps branch, and triceps long or lateral head branch to axillary nerve. J Hand Surg [Am] 2004;29(1):131–9.
17. Leechavengvongs S, Witoonchart K, Uerpairojkit C, et al. Nerve transfer to deltoid muscle using the nerve to the long head of the triceps, part II: a report of 7 cases. J Hand Surg [Am] 2003;28(4):633–8.
18. Tung T, Novak C, Mackinnon S. Nerve transfers to the biceps and brachialis branches to improve elbow flexion strength after brachial plexus injuries. J Neurosurg 2003;98(2):313–8.
19. Malessy M, Thomeer R. Evaluation of intercostal to musculocutaneous nerve transfer in reconstructive

brachial plexus surgery. J Neurosurg 1998;88: 266–71.

20. Gu Y, Xu J, Chen L, et al. Long term outcome of con-tralateral C7 transfer: a report of 32 cases. Chin Med J (Engl) 2002;115(6):866–8.

21. Gu YD, Chen DS, Zhang GM, et al. Long-term func-tional results of contralateral C7 transfer. J Reconstr Microsurg 1998;14(1):57–9.

22. Gu YD, Cai PQ, Xu F, et al. Clinical application of ip-silateral C7 nerve root transfer for treatment of C5 and C6 avulsion of brachial plexus. Microsurgery 2003;23(2):105–8.

23. Xu WD, Xu JG, Gu YD. Comparative clinic study on vascularized and nonvascularized full-length phrenic nerve transfer. Microsurgery 2005;25(1): 16–20.

24. Xu WD, Gu YD, Xu JG, et al. Full-length phrenic nerve transfer by means of video-assisted thoracic surgery in treating brachial plexus avulsion injury. Plast Reconstr Surg 2002;110(1):104–9.

25. Xu WD, Gu YD, Lu JB, et al. Pulmonary function after complete unilateral phrenic nerve transection. J Neurosurg 2005;103(3):464–7.

26. Samardzic M, Grujicic D, Antunovic V. Reinnervation of avulsed brachial plexus using spinal accessory nerve. Surg Neurol 1990;33:7–11.

27. Bertelli J, Ghizoni M. Transfer of the accessory nerve to the suprascapular nerve in brachial plexus recon-struction. J Hand Surg [Am] 2007;32:989–98.

28. Malessy M, De Rutter G, De Boer K, et al. Evaluation of suprascapular nerve neurotization after nerve graft or transfer in the treatment of brachial plexus traction lesions. J Neurosurg 2004;101:377–89.

29. Samardzic M, Rasulic L, Grujicic D. Results of nerve transfer to the musculocutaneous and axillary nerves. Neurosurgery 2000;46:93–103.

30. Samii A, Carvalho G, Samii M. Brachial plexus injury: factors affecting functional outcome in spinal acces-sory nerve transfer for the restoration of elbow flexion. J Neurosurg 2003;98:307–12.

31. Songcharoen P, Mahaisavariya B, Chotigavanich C. Spinal accessory neurotization for restoration of elbow flexion in avulsion injuries of the brachial plexus. J Hand Surg [Am] 1996;21:387–90.

32. Waikakul S, Wongtragul S, Vanadurongwan V. Res-toration of elbow flexion in brachial plexus avulsion injury: comparing spinal accessory nerve transfer with intercostal nerve transfer. J Hand Surg [Am] 1999;24:571–7.

33. Merrell G, Barrie K, Katz DL. Results of nerve transfer techniques for restoration of shoulder and elbow func-tion in the context of a meta-analysis of the English liter-ature. J Hand Surg [Am] 2001;26:303–14.

34. Colbert S, Mackinnon S. Posterior approach for dou-ble nerve transfer for restoration of shoulder function in upper brachial plexus palsy. Hand 2006;1:71–7.

35. Friedman A, Nunley J, Goldner R. Nerve transposi-tion for the restoration of elbow flexion following brachial plexus avulsion injuries. J Neurosurg 1990;72:59–64.

36. Mano Y, Nakamuro T, Tamura R. Central motor re-covery after anastomosis of the musculocutaneous and intercostal nerves following cervical root avul-sion. Ann Neurol 1995;38:15–20.

37. Okinaga S, Nagano A. Can vascularization improve the surgical outcome of the intercostal nerve transfer for traumatic brachial plexus palsy? A clinical comparison of vascularized and non-vascularized methods. Microsurgery 1999;19(4):176–80.

38. Chuang M, Chuang C, Lin I, et al. Ventilation and excercise performance after phrenic nerve and mul-tiple intercostal nerve transfers for avulsed brachial plexus injury. Chest 2005;128:3434–9.

39. Terzis J, Vekris M, Soucacos PN. Outcomes of brachial plexus reconstruction in 204 patients with devastating paralysis. Plast Reconstr Surg 1999; 104:1221–40.

40. Sungpet A, Suphachatwong C, Kawinwonggowit V. Sensory abnormalities after the seventh cervical nerve root transfer. Microsurgery 1999;19:287–8.

41. Ali Z, Meyer R, Belzberg A. Neuropathic pain after C7 spinal nerve transection in man. Pain 2002;96: 41–7.

42. Songcharoen P, Wongtrakul S, Mahaisavariya B, et al. Hemi-contralateral C7 transfer to median nerve in the treatment of root avulsion brachial plexus injury. J Hand Surg [Am] 2001;26:1058–64.

43. Liang C, Gu Y, Hu S, et al. Contralateral C7 transfer for the treatment of brachial plexus root avulsion in children—a report of 12 cases. J Hand Surg [Am] 2007;32:96–103.

44. Mcguiness C, Kay S. The pre-spinal route in contra-lateral C7 nerve root transfer for brachial plexus avulsion injuries. J Hand Surg [Br] 2002;27:159–60.

45. Dolenc VV. Intercostal neurotization of the peripheral nerves in avulsion plexus injuries. Clin Plast Surg 1984;11:143–7.

46. Narakas AO. Thoughts on neurotization or nerve transfers in irreparable nerve lesions. Clin Plast Surg 1984;11:153–9.

47. Gilbert A. Long-term evaluation of brachial plexus surgery in obstetric palsy. Hand Clin 1995;11: 583–95.

48. Brandt K, Mackinnon S. A technique for maximizing biceps recovery in brachial plexus reconstruction. J Hand Surg [Am] 1993;18:726–33.

49. Samardzic M, Grujicic D, Rasulic L, et al. Transfer of the medial pectoral nerve: myth or reality? Neurosur-gery 2002;50:1277–82.

50. Blaauw G, Slooff A. Transfer of pectoral nerves to the musculocutaneous nerve in obstetric upper brachial plexus palsy. Neurosurgery 2003;53:338–42.

51. Aszmann O, Rab M, Kamloz L, et al. The anatomy of the pectoral nerves and their significance in brachial plexus reconstruction. J Hand Surg [Am] 2000;25: 942–7.

52. Sungpet A, Suphachatwong C, Kawinwonggowit V. Surgical anatomy of bicipital branch of musculocutaneous nerve. J Med Assoc Thai 1998;81:532–5.

53. Chen Z, Xu J, Shen L, et al. Phrenic nerve conduction study in patients with traumatic brachial plexus palsy. Muscle Nerve 2001;24:1388–90.

54. Songcharoen P. Brachial plexus injury in Thailand: a report of 520 cases. Microsurgery 1995;16:35–9.

55. Luedemann W, Hamm M, Blomer U. Brachial plexus neurotization with donor phrenic nerves and its effect on pulmonary function. J Neurosurg 2002;96:523–6.

56. Leechavengvongs S, Witoonchart K, Uerpairojkit C, et al. Nerve transfer to biceps muscle using a part of the ulnar nerve in brachial plexus injury (upper arm type): a report of 32 cases. J Hand Surg [Am] 1998;23:711–6.

57. Sungpet A, Uphachatwong C, Kawinwonggowit V. Transfer of a single fascicle from the ulnar nerve to biceps muscle after avulsions of upper roots of the brachial plexus. J Hand Surg [Br] 2000;25:325–8.

58. Mackinnon SE. Preliminary results of double nerve transfer to restore elbow flexion in upper type brachial plexus palsies. Plast Reconstr Surg 2006; 118(5):1273.

59. Sungpet A, Suphachatwong C, Kawinwonggowit V. One-fascicle median nerve transfer to biceps muscle in C5 and C6 root avulsion of brachial plexus injury. Microsurgery 2003;23:10–3.

60. Ferraresi S, Garozzo D, Buffatti P. Reinnervation of the biceps in C5-7 brachial plexus avulsion injury: results after distal bypass surgery. Neurosurg Focus 2004;15:E6.

61. Nath R, Mackinnon S, Shenaq S. New nerve transfers following peripheral nerve injuries. Plastic Reconstructive Surgery 1997;4:2–11.

62. Battiston B, Lanzetta M. Reconstruction of high ulnar nerve lesions by distal double median to ulnar nerve transfer. J Hand Surg [Am] 1999;24:1185–91.

63. Novak C, Mackinnon SE. Distal anterior interosseous nerve transfer to the deep motor branch of the ulnar nerve for reconstruction of high ulnar nerve injury. J Reconstr Microsurg 2002;18(6):459–63.

64. Samardzic MM, Grujicic DM, Rasulic LG, et al. The use of thoracodorsal nerve transfer in restoration of irreparable C5 and C6 spinal nerve lesions. Br J Plast Surg 2005;58(4):541–6.

65. Novak CB, Mackinnon SE, Tung TH. Patient outcome following a thoracodorsal to musculocutaneous nerve transfer for reconstruction of elbow flexion. Br J Plast Surg 2002;55(5):416–9.

66. Brunelli GA. Sensory nerves transfers. J Hand Surg [Br] 2004;29(6):557–62.

Nerve Root Replantation

Thomas Carlstedt, PhD, MB[a,b,c,]*

KEYWORDS

- Brachial plexus injury • Spinal nerve root avulsion
- Spinal cord replantation • Functional recovery
- Pain • Plasticity

Spinal nerve root avulsion injury is a lesion where the nerves linking the spinal cord to the muscles or various sensory receptors have been torn or avulsed from the spinal cord (**Fig. 1**). This is a "longitudinal spinal cord injury," as motor and sensory fibers within the affected spinal cord segments are interrupted. The root avulsion injury is most frequent in severe brachial plexus lesions from high-energy trauma such as a motorbike accident at high speed, in which the forequarter has been violently impacted or has become dissociated from the trunk. Avulsion of at least one spinal nerve root of the brachial plexus has been estimated to occur in about 70% of all brachial plexus lesions.[1] The lower roots of the plexus, ie, C8 and T1, are more easily avulsed than the upper roots C5 to C7, because the latter are supported by ligaments at the exit foramina. Traction forces strong enough to overcome those ligaments can cause a complete C5-T1 brachial plexus avulsion injury.

Although the exact process leading to root avulsion is not completely understood, two mechanisms have been described (**Fig. 2**). The *peripheral mechanism* is a lateral or peripheral traction force onto the root and spinal nerve that, when forceful enough, pulls the root off the spinal cord and displaces the roots with the ganglia out of the spinal canal and the intervertebral foramina.[2] This is prevalent in adult trauma cases. After such a traction, the roots and the dorsal root ganglion can be found in between the scalene muscles or, even further distally, underneath the clavicle. In the *central mechanism*, the roots have been detached from the spinal cord, but the ganglion and the roots have not been displaced out of the spinal canal or the foramen. This

paradoxical situation is thought to depend on an axial rather than a lateral force occurring during a shift in the spinal cord from excessive lateral flexion of the cervical spine.[2] In that movement, the spinal cord pulls in cranial direction away from the roots that are anchored at the intervertebral foramina. This type of root avulsion is likely to occur when there has been an impact to the cervical spine, sometimes with vertebral fractures, rather than trauma to the shoulder. A mixture of peripheral and central mechanisms of root avulsion is often seen in the obstetric brachial plexus injury.

The clinical effect of the root avulsion injury is loss of movements and sensory dysfunction in the affected limb, ie, a monoplegia. Early, in many cases on the day of injury, there is a typical severe excruciating pain. It consists of two components: one is constant as dull ace and the other is intermittent as shooting severe jolts of a burning and compression sensation.[3] In about 10% of severe brachial plexus avulsion injuries there is a Brown–Sequard syndrome most likely from compromised circulation in the affected spinal cord segment. Other severe conditions may follow spinal nerve root avulsion. Spinal cord tethering or herniation through the dural defect after the root avulsions can give rise to tardy Brown–Sequard syndrome as well as myelopathy with spastic paraplegia, which has been reported to occur late after this injury.[4–7] The onset of such symptoms ranged from 6 months to 37 years after root avulsion. Adhesions and arachnoid cysts, in some cases from singular root avulsion, cause compression of the spinal cord and interference with circulation, particularly a chronic venous congestion resulting in ischemic insults. Significant

[a] Imperial College, Hammersmith Hospital, DuCane Road, London W12 0NN, UK
[b] Karolinska Institutet, Se 11883 Stockholm, Sweden
[c] University College London, Queen Square WC1N 3BG, London, UK
* Corresponding author. The PNI-Unit, The Royal National Orthopaedic Hospital, Brockley Hill, Stanmore, Middx, HA7 4LP, UK.
E-mail address: carlstedt.thomas@googlemail.com

Neurosurg Clin N Am 20 (2009) 39–50
doi:10.1016/j.nec.2008.07.020

neurosurgery.theclinics.com

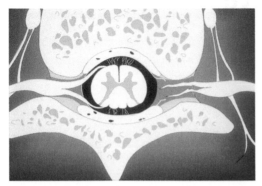

Fig. 1. Avulsion of spinal nerve roots. The connections between the CNS in the spinal cord and the extensions in the nerve roots and PNS are interrupted. (*From* Carlstedt T. Central nerve plexus injury. London: Imperial College Press; 2007; with permission.)

improvement of long tract symptoms with arrest of progression of the motor dysfunction followed surgical decompression. Other rare phenomena late after root avulsion injury includes hemosiderosis, which can be progressive and fatal.[8]

BASIC SCIENCE

At the cellular level, the root avulsion injury triggers a cascade of molecular events that leads to degeneration of nerve fibers and death of nerve cells within the spinal cord. The early response in motoneurons to avulsion means a shrinkage in size of the soma and dendrites. The number of synaptic

connections with the injured neuron is diminished, especially on the cell body and proximal dendrites.

There is a preferential loss of excitatory inputs to the motoneuron in this situation, probably leaving the cells under an inhibitory influence during the repair process.[9] These events mirror a shift in the metabolism of the severed motoneurons from subserving the role for the motoneuron as a commander of motor activity to a state where the primary goal is to survive and produce new axons. This is reflected in an increase in mRNA expression of proteins linked with cell survival such as growth factors (ie, brain derived neurotrophic factor [BDNF]) and receptors[10] as well as proteins for axonal growth (ie, growth associated protein [GAP-43]).

Motor as well as sensory neurons within the spinal cord are rapidly killed by root avulsion.[11,12] Disconnection from the periphery, meaning an interrupted supply of neutrotrophic factors together with vascular trauma leading to excitooxicity, drastically reduces the number of motoneurons up to about 90% of the normal population.[9,11] Other mechanisms to motoneuron death, such as an inflammatory response to avulsion by means of microglia activation from cytokines, has also been described.[13] Two weeks after such an injury about half of all motoneurons in the pertinent spinal cord segment have disappeared whereas an almost instantaneous 15% death of dorsal horn neurons occurs.[12] There is a further motor neuron death over time.[14] In contrast, a dorsal root avulsion does not induce any significant nerve cell death in the dorsal root ganglion.[12] Obviously the

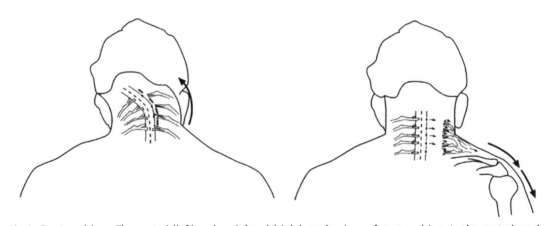

Fig. 2. Root avulsions. The central (*left*) and peripheral (*right*) mechanisms of root avulsion. In the central mechanism there is a forceful lateral flexion of the cervical spine and spinal cord (*large arrow*). There is a longitudinal shearing force that separates the roots from their attachments with the spinal cord (*small arrows*) without the roots being displaced outside the spinal canal. The spinal cord is pulled in a cranial direction in relation to the spine, whereas the roots are held by their attachments to the spine at the intervertebral foramina. The loose suspension of the shoulder girdle makes the brachial plexus particularly susceptible to traction injury when there is a trauma that separates the shoulder from the neck (*large arrows*). Root avulsions with displacements of the roots outside the spinal canal (*small arrows*) occur if the force is of significant magnitude. (*From* Carlstedt T. Central nerve plexus injury. London: Imperial College Press; 2007; with permission.)

central but not the peripheral sensory neuron is more sensitive to root trauma. The loss of dorsal horn neurons is of course of importance for the development of the classical brachial plexus avulsion pain.

The recent development and gain in knowledge from studies of molecular biology has demonstrated the importance in timing of repair of nerve injuries. One month after injury the expressions of growth factors and their receptors have already declined to the extent that outcome of repair is less favorable than if done immediately after the injury (for review see Gordon and colleagues).[15] With regard to root avulsion injury, time-dependent neuron death adds to the urgency in reconstructing these injuries as replanting the avulsed ventral root to some extent maintains the population of spinal cord neurons.

The spinal cord injury that follows from root avulsion can today be repaired with a functional outcome in humans.[16–21] The surgical strategy is based and developed from a long series of laboratory experiments. The basic requirements for regeneration of function after a spinal nerve root avulsion injury are the survival of nerve cells situated close to the injury and the regrowth of new nerve fibers along a trajectory consisting of central nervous (CNS) growth-inhibitory tissue in the spinal cord and peripheral nervous (PNS) growth-promoting tissue in nerves. This is the first example of a spinal cord lesion that can be treated surgically leading to restoration of activity and alleviation of pain (for a full description, see Carlstedt).[16]

ASSESSMENTS
Clinical

The "classical" history of a brachial plexus avulsion injury is that from patients involved in a motorcycle accident where the forequarter has been impacted resulting in a monoplegia. The patient is often able to describe the typical root avulsion pain as a constant dull, crushing, or burning pain with superimposed lightening jolts of severe sharp pain shooting down the arm.

On inspection, a Bernard-Horner sign suggests but is not a proof of avulsion of the lower roots to the plexus. Bruising and swelling at the base of the neck are ominous signs of a lesion of the longitudinal neurovascular structures.

Examination can reveal spared muscle function, but activity in the serratus anterior muscle is possible in spite of a complete brachial plexus avulsion injury. Some fascicles to the long thoracic nerve can be spared at the C5 root, although the roots are found pulled out of the foramen. The brachial plexus can, if in situ, be palpated as a ridge

just lateral to the sternocleidomastoid muscle. Tapping on this site can elicit a sharp electric sensation shooting down the arm, ie, the Tinel's sign, if there are some root or nerve stumps still in continuity with the spinal cord. In cases of a complete brachial plexus avulsion injury there is no Tinel's sign to be found, which of course is a bad sign.

Ancillary

Without any ancillary examinations, it can be initially assumed that the patient has a total brachial plexus avulsion injury if no Tinel's sign can be proved in a patient with a complete paralysis, a Bernard-Horner sign, and typical avulsion pain. Electrophysiology is of little value in the immediate posttraumatic period. It is 2 to 3 weeks later when typical denervation signs, ie, positive sharp waves and fibrillations, become obvious in the affected muscles. The presence of a sensory nerve action potential (SNAP), together with loss of sensation is, however, a useful sign of root avulsion, as the sensory neurons in the avulsed dorsal root ganglion will be alive and conducting distally but not centrally for perception.

Radiographs of the neck and upper thorax give valuable information regarding fractures and the possibility of cervical spine instability. Fractures of the transverse processes are often associated with avulsion injury to the pertinent spinal nerve roots and traumatic insult to the vertebral artery. Fracture dislocation of the first rib indicates a severe proximal or intraspinal lesion to the lower trunk of the plexus and to the subclavian artery. A raised hemidiaphragm on a chest radiograph reveals a most proximal C5 lesion.

Magnetic resonance imaging (MRI) is at present not optimal for considering individual roots.[22] Myelography followed by computerized tomography (CT) appears still to be the current imaging of choice for the assessment of roots;[23] however, it does not allow a full assessment of C8 and T1 roots because of beam-hardening artifacts from the shoulder. False or overdiagnosis of root avulsions is possible and the outcome could be difficult to understand in cases of severe contrast leakage.

SURGERY
The Exposure

The patient is in a "strict" lateral position.[24] The head is supported in a Mayfield clamp with the neck slightly flexed toward the opposite side (**Fig. 3**). The head-up position of the operating table is used to prevent venous congestion, particularly of the epidural veins. During the procedure, the operating table's tilting facilities can be used

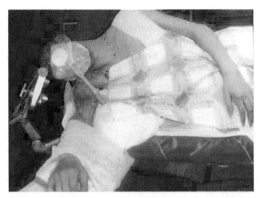

Fig. 3. Patient in a lateral position with head fixed in a Mayfield clamp and shoulder pulled down by Elastoplast. Skin incision is indicated.

when going from medial to lateral exposures of the brachial plexus. A skin incision from the jugulum into the posterior triangle of the neck toward and passing the spinous process of the C5 vertebra is performed (see **Fig. 3**). Platysma and skin flaps are raised and held either by stay sutures or a thyroid retractor. Dissections first are performed in the posterior triangle of the neck of the injured extraspinal part of the brachial plexus and the spinal accessory nerve as it emerges from the posterior aspect of the sternocleidomastoid muscle (**Fig. 4**). The accessory nerve can be cut as distal

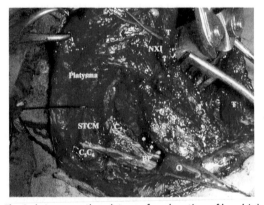

Fig. 4. Intraoperative picture of exploration of brachial plexus. The platysma has been elevated and the sternocleidomastoid muscle, the scalenei (S) and the trapezius (T) muscles are indicated. The omohyoid (O) muscle has been divided. The upper nerve roots, C5-C7, have been avulsed from the spinal cord. Asterisks indicate the empty foramina. A sling is applied around the accessory nerve (NXI). Retractors in the posterior part of the wound to expose the cervical spine. (*From* Carlstedt T, Anand P, Hallin R, et al. Spinal nerve root repair and replantation of avulsed ventral roots into the spinal cord after brachial plexus injury. J Neurosurg (Spine 2) 2000;93:237–47; with permission.)

as possible to be used later for transfer to the suprascapular nerve.

Endoscopy

When there are avulsions and the spinal nerve and roots have been pulled out from the spinal and intervertebral canal, it is possible to introduce an endoscope through the empty foramen. A small 2 mm in diameter joint arthroscope has been used. The lower foramina, ie, the C7-T1 intervertebral canal, are best suited for this maneuver as they are larger than the foramina above and do not contain the vertebral vessels (**Fig. 5**).With this technique, more information regarding remaining intradural root stumps or full root avulsions can be gained than through ancillary investigations (ie, electrophysiology or CT-myelography), particularly regarding the lower roots to the brachial plexus without proceeding to a full inspection after a laminectomy.

The second part of the dissection is to reach the cervical spine in the posterior part of the incision. No further skin incision is needed to perform this dissection. The posterior tubercles of the transverse processes of C4 to C7 can be palpated, and they are followed in the dissection through a connective tissue plane between the levator scapula and the posterior and medial scalene muscles (**Fig. 6**). The longissimus muscle deep to this plane must be split longitudinally to expose the posterior tubercles of the transverse processes and the hemilaminae (see **Fig. 6**). The paravertebral muscles are detached from the hemilaminae and pushed dorsomedially. After a standard hemilaminectomy taking away the medial part of processes for the facet joints using drills or rongeurs and breaching the periosteum (which could be confused with the dura mater), hemostasis of epidural veins, which laterally can cause irritating bleedings, is achieved. Sometimes a rent in the dura mater has been caused by the avulsion trauma and cerebrospinal fluid (CSF) starts to leak before the dura has been formally opened. The dura mater is incised longitudinally and stay sutures applied (**Fig. 7**). The denticulate ligaments that are preserved are cut from their lateral attachments. Stay sutures are applied to the part of the denticulate ligament that runs along the side of the spinal cord to gently rotate the cord (see **Fig. 7**). With this approach and with the help of the stay sutures in the denticulate ligament, it is possible to reach to the anterior aspect of the spinal cord at the ventral root exit zones. At this stage it is possible to see if the roots have been completely avulsed and displaced outside

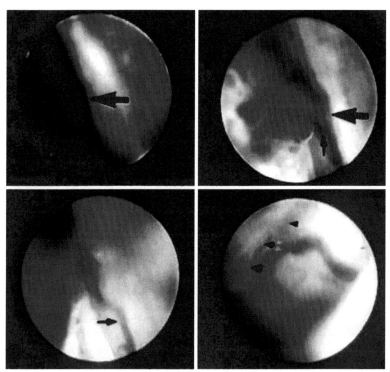

Fig. 5. Endoscopy of cervical spinal cord through empty intervertebral foramina after brachial plexus avulsion injury. Top left: at the external foramen (*arrow*). Top right: blood vessel (*arrow*) within the canal. Lower right: view of the spinal cord with blood vessel (*arrow*) on its surface. Lower right: arrows indicate site of ventral root avulsion. (*From* Carlstedt T. Central nerve plexus injury. London: Imperial College Press; 2007; with permission.)

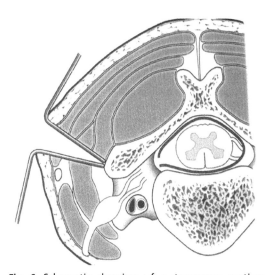

Fig. 6. Schematic drawing of a transverse section through the lower part of the neck illustrating the lateral approach to the cervical spine. The nerve roots have been avulsed from the spinal cord and the subdural space. (*From* Carlstedt T, Anand P, Hallin R, et al. Spinal nerve root repair and replantation of avulsed ventral roots into the spinal cord after brachial plexus injury. J Neurosurg (Spine 2) 2000;93:237–47; with permission.)

the spinal canal (see **Fig. 7**) or still remain within the subdural space in the spinal canal.

The Repair

Detached nerve roots can be retrieved through the intervertebral foramen if the surgery is performed within days after the accident. This is done with great care using a tube or a catheter, avoiding injury to the vertebral vessels (see **Fig. 7**). This is not possible if the surgery is delayed more than 2 weeks, as the displaced roots will be scarred and the intervertebral foramen sealed by scar tissue. In some cases, the avulsed roots can be situated within the subdural space allowing for a direct replantation. In most cases, however, nerve grafting is the only possibility to reconnect the spinal cord to the avulsed roots (**Fig. 8**). The nerve graft (taken preferentially from the superficial radial, the medial cutaneous nerve of the ipsilateral forearm, or the sural nerve) is split into separate fascicles for two to four different spinal cord segments and introduced to a depth of about 1 to 2 mm by means of a probe, leaving another 2 mm of white matter to the ventral horn and the motoneuron pool. Useful in this maneuver is a small Rhoton instrument in the shape of a hockey stick, the

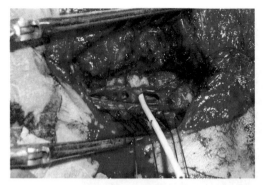

Fig. 7. Intraoperative picture. The partly torn dura has been opened. No remaining roots are seen in the subdural space. A catheter is introduced through C7 intervertebral canal, with the other end in the posterior triangle of the neck ready to apply nerve grafts. (*From* Carlstedt T. Central nerve plexus injury. London: Imperial College Press; 2007; with permission.)

"blade" of which being 1 to 2 mm in length can be used as a depth gauge when implanting the root or the nerve graft. The position of the implanted grafts is retained by glue (Tisseel). Stitching the graft to the pia mater can also be done, but is difficult. In case of root ruptures the nerve graft is directly apposed to the trimmed end of the ventral root stump. The nerve grafts are pulled trough the intervertebral foramen for C7 or C8 spinal nerves (see **Fig. 8**). If the foramen is blocked, the grafts are passed through the incision in the dura and outside the vertebral canal. The grafts are connected to the avulsed roots in the posterior triangle of the neck where they have been displaced by the traction trauma. During the intraspinal procedure, spinal cord monitoring of motor tract function (MEP) together with somatosensory-evoked potential (SSEP) is performed. The dura is not usually closed but the opening in the dura is covered by artificial dura or a vein patch and Tisseel glue. A lumbar drain could be applied for about 1 week to prevent the development of CSF leakage. The patient is mobilized after a week but the arm is kept in a sling for a total of 6 weeks.

Outcome

Motor recovery

Most patients started to recover muscle function within 1 year after the injury, seen as muscle twitches (Medical Research Council [MRC] grade 1/5) in the pectoral muscle.[17,18,21] Muscle activity returned first in shoulder muscles followed by upper arm muscles about a year later and in a few cases as far distally as to one or two forearm muscles during the third year. There was an eventual increase in power in shoulder girdle muscles, ie, serratus anterior, pectoral, and supraspinatus muscles to a significant power, in many cases reaching a normal magnitude ie, MRC 4-5/5 (**Fig. 9**).

There was less power in upper arm muscles that never reached a normal but a useful level ie, MRC 3-4/5. Obviously there is not a specific motoneuron to the original target regeneration. The regrowing new axons try to reinnervate the first possible muscle target, which are the shoulder muscles.

Consequently, there is less reinnervation in more distal muscles (**Fig. 10**). Muscle power in some forearm muscles reached only about MRC 2/5, ie, not functional. However, spinal cord replantation after a complete avulsion injury in a preadolescent boy resulted in recovery of hand function together with useful activity in shoulder and arm.[21] Intrinsic muscle recovery was verified by electromyography (EMG) and he developed a transverse palm and pinch grip (**Fig. 11**) that is useful in many daily

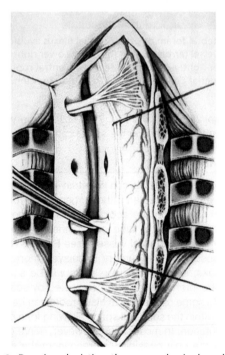

Fig. 8. Drawing depicting the exposed spinal cord after a lateral approach and hemilaminectomy. The dura mater has been opened, and by stay sutures in the denticulate ligament, the spinal cord has been slightly rotated for access to its ventral part. Through slits in the pia mater and the spinal cord surface, nerve grafts are implanted superficially into the spinal cord. (*From* Carlstedt T, Birch R. Management of acute peripheral nerve injuries. In: Winn R, editor. Youmans neurological surgery. Philadelphia: Saunders; 2004; with permission.)

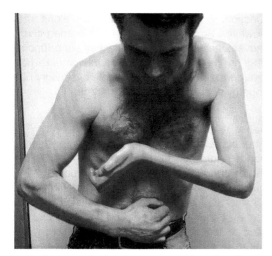

Fig. 9. Photograph showing return of function 3 years after replantation surgery in a case of complete brachial plexus avulsion injury. Good muscle activity in shoulder and upper arm muscles with some muscle contraction in radial forearm muscles.

activities as well as making it possible for him to play drums with the affected hand.

The final muscle power in major proximal muscles of MRC Grade 4/5 was noted only in patients who had been operated within a moth or earlier after the trauma. Patients operated late recovered very little or nonuseful muscle power. This is consistent with the experimental findings of time-dependent motoneuron loss after avulsion injury.[14] Moreover, motoneuron programs for repair are available for a limited period after injury and are effective only if the severed axons are offered a conduit for regrowth.[15] When reconstruction is delayed, the growth-associated genes are downregulated and the neurons become atrophic or die. With delay of repair there is also an impairment of Schwann cell ability to support regeneration[25] as well as the deterioration of the denervated muscles.[14] In spite of a considerable motoneuron loss from the root avulsion trauma, there was a consistent recovery of muscle power, which in proximal muscle groups was near to normal. Of importance

in this recovery is obviously the ability of surviving motoneurons to establish larger than normal motor units that can compensate for an 80% loss of neurons.[26]

Magnetic cortical stimulation demonstrated and verified the clinical observation of connectivity from motor cortex to the previously denervated muscles through the reconstructed spinal cord–peripheral nerve trajectories. The latency of the muscle response was generally longer than in the intact arm, indicating that the regenerated nerve fibers were not fully developed and less myelinated than on the normal side.

Severe co-contractions or synkinesis between agonistic and antagonistic muscles such as biceps and triceps occurred in most patients. Nonspecific recruitment of motoneurons through the implanted PNS conduit and lack of guidance or misdirection of axons causes aberrant muscle reinnervation.

Inappropriate muscle reinnervation applies also to the phrenic motoneurons regenerating to arm muscles after replantation of ventral root or PNS graft, causing respiratory-related limb muscle contractions. This peculiar type of synergism was noted in some patients where the implantation into the C5 spinal cord segment provoked spontaneous contractions of arm muscles in synchrony with respiration, ie, "the breathing arm" phenomenon.[21] Muscle contractions synchronous with spontaneous inspiration were generally related to recovery of volitional function but could also occur in muscle without voluntary function, ie, MRC 0/5. Different combinations of muscles mainly in the C5 myotome showed this activity, ie, pectoral, deltoid, biceps, and triceps muscles.

The occurrence of the breathing arm phenomenon in patients after complete brachial plexus avulsion injury with subsequent spinal cord replantation is caused by CNS or spinal cord regeneration. The anatomic background to this is the caudal part of the phrenic motoneuron nucleus is extending into the C5 segment. These neurons are situated most medially in the ventral horn and after reimplantation of an avulsed ventral root or

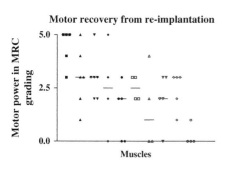

Motor recovery from re-implantation

- ■ Serratus anterior
- ▲ Pectoralis Maj (Cl)
- ▼ Pectoralis Maj (St)
- ◆ Supraspinatus
- ● Infraspinatus
- ◻ Latissimus dorsi
- △ Deltoid
- ▽ Biceps
- ◇ Triceps
- ○ Flexor carpi radialis

Fig. 10. Diagram showing recovery of muscle power after spinal cord replantation of avulsed ventral roots. Power decreases in distal direction. (*From* Carlstedt T. Central nerve plexus injury. London: Imperial College Press; 2007; with permission.)

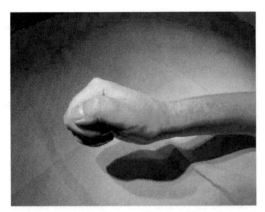

Fig. 11. Recovered transverse hand and pinch grip in a preadolescent boy who sustained a complete brachial plexus avulsion injury. Hand function returned 3 years after replantation surgery.

a peripheral nerve conduit into this segment phrenic motoneurons are recruited to extend axons along the peripheral nerves to the arm rather than into the phrenic nerve to the diaphragm (**Fig. 12**).

The lack of sensory reconnection with the pertinent spinal cord segment after intraspinal repair means lack of muscle proprioception. In such a situation without la afference there is no reciprocal inhibition of antagonistic muscles. A mass movement without the ability to activate individual joints is a sign of supraspinal-led activity without proprioceptive feedback and to some extent this deficient afferent control over muscle function leads to co-contractions. Some degree of muscle proprioception would be necessary for good muscle function. A central motor program alone may, however, be sufficient to execute learned simple movements such as elbow flexion. Limb function and, in particular, purposeful movements have been described in a rare example of sensory neuropathy with loss of muscle afferents.[27]

Sensory recovery

After complete C5-T1 root avulsion injury, sensation is poor after this type of surgery, where only motor conduits have been reconstructed.[20] Pinprick sensation was usually subnormal in the C5, diminished in C6, and absent in C7-T1 dermatomes. Sense of joint position could be appreciated at the shoulder but also at the elbow. The return of some sensory function such as proprioception, temperature, and pain in avulsed dermatomes is unexpected and difficult to explain, as only the ventral roots have been reconnected to the pertinent spinal cord segments. Whether this function depends on extensions of new processes from dorsal horn neurons along the implanted ventral root or whether it is related to collaterals from adjacent spinal cord segments is at the present unknown.

Sensory stimulation within the avulsed dermatomes was mostly perceived abnormally and or experienced at remote sites as referred sensation.[20] Intraspinal afferent sprouting producing terminal fields extending into spinal cord segments that have sustained root avulsion and deafferentation[28] could explain such phenomena as referrals of sensation from the region of the neck to the hand or the other way around. Classical "right way" referral of sensation when sensory

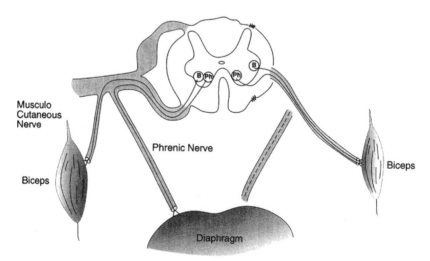

Fig. 12. Diagram showing erroneous spinal cord regeneration of axons from the phrenic motoneuron nucleus in the spinal cord, causing the "breathing arm" phenomenon. Ph, phrenic motoneurons; B, biceps motoneurons. (*From* Carlstedt T. Central nerve plexus injury. London: Imperial College Press; 2007; with permission.)

stimulation of the hand was perceived at the trunk, neck, or face or "wrong way" referral of sensation from the face, neck ,or trunk to the affected arm occurred (**Fig. 13**).[20,29] In the early weeks after injury and repair there was referral of sensation from central parts of the body, even viscera to the affected arm.

Pain

The severe pain sustained by patients suffering from brachial plexus injury is typical[20,30] and is presumed to be caused by the generation of abnormal activity in deafferented spinal cord segments.[31] There is a correlation between number of roots avulsed and severity of pain.[20] Remarkable is that in patients with complete avulsion injury to the brachial plexus followed by ventral root replantation there is reduction of pain correlated to return of muscle activity rather than other qualities of function.[20,29] In patients who had recovery of motor function limited to the upper part of the extremity there is persisting pain in the hand. In a case of a preadolescent boy with complete plexus avulsion and after replantation there was motor recovery in all parts of the arm and the hand. There was a complete alleviation of the severe pain when motor function recovered. The mechanism behind this is difficult to explain, but selective loss of motor fibers after ventral rhizotomy can provoke pain in animals[32,33] and

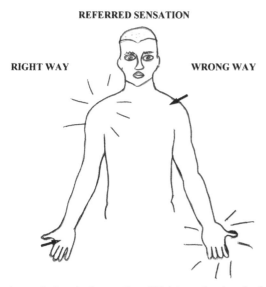

REFERRED SENSATION

RIGHT WAY   WRONG WAY

Fig. 13. Referral of sensation. "Right way" referral of sensation: Touching the hand is perceived in the upper part of the trunk because of growth of transferred nerves into the hand. "Wrong way" referral of sensation: Touching an area at the base of the neck or the face is perceived in the hand because of cortex plasticity.

humans.[34] In some patients there was allodynia to mechanical and/or thermal stimulation.[20] The area of allodynia was at the border zone of affected and unaffected dermatomes, usually at the border of T1 and T2 dermatomes, at the back of the elbow. The allodynia was not bothersome and minor in comparison with the deafferentation pain.

Plasticity

In cases of muscle co-contraction there was an eventual tendency for one of the antagonistic muscles—the biceps or the triceps—to dominate and for the antagonistic to be functionally suppressed indicating a degree of plasticity, but isolated contraction in individual muscles could still not be performed. Synkinesis and breathing arm phenomena were noted in long-term follow-up indicating a stationary condition.[21] In general there was no sign of spinal cord plasticity to modulate muscle activity to become purely voluntary. The lack of plasticity as well as methods to correct the misdirection of motoneurons is known also from children with obstetric brachial plexus injury.[35] In experimental studies, this lack of modification of spinal motoneurons connected inappropriately even in the young or immature animal has been documented.[36] There seems to be an inability of motor programs to change when innervating a new target and that motor circuits are usually maintained, even after the motoneurons innervate a foreign muscle.[37]

Contrary to the lack of spinal cord plasticity is the well established fact that supraspinal parts of the central nervous system can become reorganized after deafferentation, which may explain the "wrong way" referred sensations (see **Fig. 13**).[38] Plasticity and reorganization of the somatosensory cortex, which may underlie referred sensation, have been demonstrated by imaging studies.[38,39] The hand, trunk, and face cortical representations are situated adjacent to each other. After dennervation of the hand, expansion of inputs from the face or trunk into the former hand territory can occur. Reorganization of the somatosensory cortex by expansion of the adjacent sensory area of the cortex area may explain referred sensation, but larger scale reorganization could also occur in different levels, including the thalamus.[40]

The "right way" of referral of sensation (see **Fig. 13**) appears as an early sign of recovery. It seems as if cortical circuits within the somatosensory system are not easily corrected for deafferentation and eventual misdirectional growth of sensory fibers can occur. The "wrong way" referral of sensation (see **Fig. 13**) on the other hand indicates plasticity rather than recovery. This is obvious in patients who even a long time after surgery have not developed sensation in the hand but perceive sensation in the hand when the neck, trunk, or face is touched. This phenomenon could occur early after the injury, suggesting unmasking of preexisting connections.[41] Intracortical sprouting could be the reason for later-appearing "wrong way" referral of sensation.[38]

Cortical reorganization has been correlated with severity of neuropathic pain.[42] There is no relationship between alleviation of pain and referral of sensation in these patients, although both phenomena are thought to be due to plasticity in the central nervous system.[20] Instead, there is correlation between pain alleviation and motor recovery. Successful motor recovery could lead to reestablishment of normal inhibitory processes that reveres the cortical process leading to pain.

Border zone allodynia could depend on abnormally sensitized peripheral nociceptic fibers that induce secondary changes in reorganization of the dorsal horn and central processing, leading to spinal cord hyperexcitability and pain.[43,44] The intact nociceptors of the adjacent uninjured spinal nerves may acquire abnormal spontaneous activity and chemical sensitivity may play a role in creating, or maintaining, an abnormal pain state.[34,45]

COMMENTS

The root avulsion injury is a spinal cord injury that interrupts defined populations of neurons, ie, the "final common pathway" for motor command and the sensory pathway from the peripheral sensory neurons. Patients with such spinal cord injuries from brachial or lumbosacral plexus injuries including cauda equina lesions can recover function from the reimplantation spinal cord surgery. This relatively less complicated injury compared with a "classical" transverse spinal cord lesion is obviously advantageous regarding chances for recovery.

Spinal cord surgery to restore connectivity after spinal nerve root avulsion injury can recover function and alleviate pain, as well as rescue spinal cord nerve cells and reestablish spinal cord circuits. In my opinion, this surgical technique is therefore today the most promising treatment in cases of longitudinal spinal cord or root avulsion injury. This strategy has encouraging prospects for future treatment of brachial and lumbosacral plexus injuries and possibly the most caudal transverse spinal cord injury, ie, conus medullaris injury. A transverse lesion of the conus medullaris would affect mostly the lower motoneurons and CNS parts of the peripheral sensory neurons together with nervous control over bladder and bowel function. A transverse caudal spinal cord injury at a conus level has therefore many similarities with the root avulsion or the longitudinal type of spinal cord injury and could in the future be considered for similar type of surgical strategy. Avulsed roots could be implanted cranial to the site of the transverse spinal cord lesion to reverse lower extremity paralysis with return of locomotion and reinnervate pelvic targets to reverse bladder and bowel dysfunction.

The original observations in laboratory experiments have taken a long time to become applied to human clinical practice. At present, the shortcomings of this technique are proportionate to the delay of surgery with death of nerve cells and incomplete and unpredictable sensimotor recovery. To reach further, to recover useful sensory-motor function and to alleviate pain, it is of course necessary to pursue research and development of basic and clinical science. Surgical and imaging refinements are also obligatory to achieve a full or near normal functional restitution after brachial plexus and lumbosacral plexus avulsion injuries with minimal risks and efforts for the patient. A number of already available pharmaceutical substances, molecular products, and cellular therapies will be applied in the future to continue the achievement of recovery of injuries at the spinal cord surface but also to help in finding cure for the more complete spinal cord injuries (for further reading see Carlstedt).[16]

REFERENCES

1. Narakas AO. Lesions found when operating traction injuries of the brachial plexus. Clin Neurol Neurosurg 1993;95(Suppl):S56–64.
2. Sunderland S, Bradley KC. Stress–strain phenomenon in human spinal nerve roots. Brain 1961;84:120–4.
3. Wynn Parry CB. Pain in avulsion lesions of the brachial plexus. Pain 1980;9:41–53.
4. Penfield W. Late spinal paralysis after avulsion of the brachial plexus. J bone Joint Surg 1949;31B:40–1.
5. Cilluffo JM, Miller RH. Posttraumatic arachniod diverticula. Acta Neurochir (Wien) 1980;54:77–87.
6. Walter H, Fairholm D. Giant intraspinal pseudomeningoceles cause delayed neurological dysfunction after brachial plexus injury: report of three cases. Neurosurg 2000;46:1245–9.
7. DaSilva VR, Al-Gahtany M, Midha R, et al. Upper thoracic spinal cord herniation after traumatic nerve root avulsion [case report and review of literature]. J Neurosurg (Spine3) 2003;99:306–9.
8. Cohen-Gadol AA, Krauss WE, Spinner RJ. Delayed central nervous system superficial siderosis

following brachial plexus avulsion injury. Neurosurg Focus 2004;16(5):14.

9. Lindå H, Risling M, Cullheim S. "Dendraxons" in regenerating motoneurons in the cat: do dendrites generate new axons after central axotomy? Brain Res 1985;358:329–33.

10. Piehl F, Hammarberg H, Tabar G, et al. Changes in the mRNA expression patterns with special reference to calcitonin gene-related peptide, after axonal injuries in rat motoneuron depend on age and time of injury. Exp Brain Res 1998;119:191–204.

11. Koliatsos VE, Price WL, Pardo CA, et al. Ventral root avulsion: an experimental model of death of adult motor neurons. J Comp Neurol 1994;342:35–44.

12. Chew DJ, Leinster VHL, Sakthithasan M, et al. Cell death after dorsal root injury. Neuroscience Letters 2008;433:231–4.

13. Olsson T, Lundberg C, Lidman O, et al. Genetic regulation of nerve avulsion-induced spinal cord inflammation. Ann N Y Acad Sci 2001;917:186–96.

14. Bergerot A, Shortland PJ, Anand P, et al. Co-treatment with riluzole and GDNF is necessary for functional recovery after ventral root avulsion injury. Exp Neurol 2004;187:359–66.

15. Gordon T, Sulaiman O, Boyd JG. Experimental strategies to promote functional recovery after peripheral nerve injuries. J Peripher Nerv Syst 2003;8:236–50.

16. Carlstedt T. Central nerve plexus injury. London: Imperial College Press; 2007.

17. Carlstedt T, Grane P, Hallin R, et al. Return of function after spinal cord implantation of avulsed spinal nerve roots. Lancet 1995;346:1323–5.

18. Carlstedt T, Anand P, Hallin R, et al. Spinal nerve root repair and reimplantation of avulsed ventral roots into the spinal cord after brachial plexus injury. J Neurosurg (Spine 2) 2000;93:237–47.

19. Carlstedt T, Anand P, Htut M, et al. Restoration of hand function and so called "breathing arm" after intraspinal repair of C5-T1 brachial plexus avulsion injury. Neurosurg Focus 2004;16(5):1–5.

20. Htut M, Misra VP, Anand P, et al. Pain phenomena and sensory recovery following brachial plexus avulsion injury and surgical repairs. J Hand Surg 2006; 31B(6)):596–605.

21. Htut M, Misra VP, Anand P, et al. Motor recovery and the breathing arm after brachial plexus surgical repairs, including reimplantation of avulsed spinal roots into the spinal cord. J Hand Surg 2007; 32E(2)):170–8.

22. Hems T, Birch R, Carlstedt T. The role of magnetic resonance imaging in the management of traction injuries to the adult brachial plexus. J Hand Surg 1999;24B(5)):550–5.

23. Belzberg AJ, Dorsi MJ, Storm PB, et al. Surgical repair of brachial plexus injury: a multinational survey of experienced peripheral nerve surgeons. J Neurosurg 2004;101:365–76.

24. Kratimentos GP, Crockard HA. The far lateral approach for ventrally placed foramen magnum and upper cervical spine tumours. Br J Neurosurg 1993;7:129–40.

25. Sulaiman OA, Midha R, Munro CA, et al. Chronic Schwann cell denervation and the presence of a sensory nerve reduce motor axon regeneration. Exp Neurol 2003;176:342–54.

26. Gordon T, Yang JF, Ayer K, et al. Recovery potentials of muscle after partial denervation: a comparison between rats and humans. Brain Res Bull 1993;30: 477–82.

27. Cole JD, Sedgewick EM. The perception of force and movement in a man without large myelinated sensory afferents below the neck. J Physiol 1992; 449:503–15.

28. McMahon S, Kett-White R. Sprouting of peripherally regenerating primary sensory neurons in the adult central nervous system. J Comp Neurol 1991;304: 307–15.

29. Berman J, Birch R, Anand P. Pain following human brachial plexus injury with spinal cord root avulsion and the effect of surgery. Pain 1998;75:199–207.

30. Frazier CH, Skillern PG. Supraclavicular subcutaneous lesion of the brachial plexus not associated with skeletal injuries. JAMA 1911;57:1957–63.

31. Ovelman-Levitt J. Abnormal physiology of the dorsal horn as related to the deafferentation syndrome. Appl Neurophysiol 1988;51:104–16.

32. Sheth R, Dorsi MJ, Li Y, Murison BB, et al. Mechanical hyperalgesia after an L5 ventral rhizotomy or an L5 ganglionectomy in the rat. Pain 2002;96: 63–72.

33. Wu G, Ringkamp M, Murison BB, et al. Degeneration of myelinated efferent fibres induces spontaneous activity in uninjured C-fibre afferents. J Nephrol 2002;22:7746–53.

34. Ali Z, Meyer RA, Belzberg AJ. Neuropathic pain after C7 spinal nerve transaction in man. Pain 2002;96: 41–7.

35. Roth G. Reinnervation dans la paralysie plexulaire brachaile obstetrical. J Nurs Scholarsh 1983;58: 103–15.

36. Gordon T, Stein RB, Thomas C. Innervation and function of hind-limb muscles in the cat after cross-union of the tibial and peroneal nerves. J Philos 1986;374:429–41.

37. Gruart A, Streppel M, Guntinas-Lichius O, et al. Motoneuron adaptability to new motor tasks following two types of facial-facial anastomosis in cats. Brain 2003;126:115–33.

38. Kaas JH, Merzenich MM, Killackey HP. The reorganization of somatosensory cortex following peripheral nerve damage in adult and developing mammals. Annu Rev Neurosci 1983;6:325–56.

39. Kew JJ, Halligan PW, Marshall JC, et al. Abnormal access of axial vibrotactile input to deafferented

somatosensory cortex in human upper limb amputees. J Neurophysiol 1997;77:2753–64.

40. Banati RB, Cagnin A, Brooks DJ, et al. Long-term trans-
synaptic glial responses in the human thalamus after
peripheral nerve injury. Neuroreport 2001;12:3439–42.

41. Borsook D, Becerra L, Fishman S, et al. Acute plasticity in the human somatosensory cortex following
amputation. Neuroreport 1998;9:1013–7.

42. Floor H, Elbert T, Knecht S, et al. Phantom-limb
pain as a perceptual correlate of cortical
reorganization following arm amputation. Nature
1995;375:482–94.

43. Baron R. Neuropathic pain. The long path from
mechanism to mechanism-based treatment. Anaes-
thetist 2000;49:373–86.

44. Baron R. Peripheral neuropathic pain: from mechanisms to symptoms. Clin J Pain 2000;16:
S12–20.

45. Campbell JN. Nerve lesions and the generation of
pain. Muscle Nerve 2001;24:1261–73.

Late Reconstruction for Brachial Plexus Injury

Brian T. Carlsen, MD[a], Allen T. Bishop, MD[b],
Alexander Y. Shin, MD[b],*

KEYWORDS

- Brachial plexus injury • Late reconstruction
- Free-functioning muscle transfers • Tendon transfers

Traumatic brachial plexus injuries are devastating and management is complex. The best approach is multidisciplinary and best managed at centers with expertise in diagnosis, treatment, and rehabilitation of these patients. Brachial plexus surgery can be divided into early and late reconstructive procedures. Early reconstruction focuses on repair or reconstruction of the nerves of the brachial plexus. These procedures include direct repair, neurolysis for scar compression, nerve grafting, and nerve transfers. However, these procedures are effective only when performed within 6 to 9 months from injury as a time-dependent change occurs in the motor endplate, which diminishes reinnervation potential.[1–10]

Axonal regeneration occurs at a rate of 1 to 2.5 mm/d in humans.[11] Therefore, muscles that are 50 cm or more from the site of repair may take more than 1 year for reinnervation. If muscle reinnervation by nerve repair or transfer is attained within 1 year, some function, especially of proximal muscles, can be restored.[12] However, at 1 year, muscle loses some of its contractibility, and at 18 to 24 months, irreversible changes develop in the motor endplate and the muscle becomes nonresponsive to neural stimuli. This fundamental principle explains why outcomes are favorable for nerve repair or transfer for restoration of shoulder and elbow function, and results are much less favorable for hand and wrist function.[8,13,14]

Late (or secondary) reconstruction is considered when patients either (1) present outside the optimal time window for nerve reconstruction or nerve transfer or (2) have incomplete function after primary reconstruction.[15] The priorities for restoring function in the delayed case remain the same and include, in order of importance, elbow flexion, shoulder abduction and/or stability, hand sensation, wrist extension and finger flexion, wrist flexion and finger extension, and finally, intrinsic hand function. Because of the limitations on nerve regeneration and distant muscle reinnervation, restoration of intrinsic hand function is not possible. The main focus in secondary reconstruction should be restoration of elbow flexion and shoulder function or stability. Elbow flexion can be restored through tendon transfers or pedicled muscle transfers of functioning muscles (ie, bipolar pectoralis muscle transfer or latissimus dorsi muscle transfer).[16–21]

However, often a pan-plexus injury is present and muscles that are functioning or of adequate strength are not available to transfer. In these cases, use of a free-functioning muscle transfer (FFMT) is indicated. Late reconstruction of shoulder stability may be achieved through muscle or tendon transfers,[18,22–24] which typically provide stability with minimal restoration of motion, or with shoulder arthrodesis.[25–27] Depending on the situation, rudimentary hand function (prehension) may be restored with a single or second FFMT.[15] Finally, wrist and selective hand and thumb arthrodesis may also improve function. Other procedures, such as tendon transfers for wrist extension or thumb opposition, wrist arthrodesis, thumb axis arthrodesis, bone-block opponensplasty, or finger

[a] Mayo Clinic, Division of Hand Surgery, 200 1st Street South West, Rochester, MN 55905, USA
[b] Mayo Clinic, Department of Orthopaedic Surgery, Division of Hand Surgery, 200 1st Street South West, Rochester, MN 55905, USA
* Corresponding author.
E-mail address: shin.alexander@mayo.edu (A. Shin).

Neurosurg Clin N Am 20 (2009) 51–64
doi:10.1016/j.nec.2008.07.021

neurosurgery.theclinics.com

joint arthrodesis, may improve function in selected cases, but are beyond the scope of this review.

FREE-FUNCTIONING MUSCLE TRANSFER FOR ELBOW FUNCTION

Microneurovascular FFMT involves the surgical transfer of a muscle and its neurovascular pedicle to a new location to assume a new function. This muscle is powered by transferring a viable motor nerve to the nerve of the FFMT and restoring the circulation of the transferred muscle with microsurgical anastomosis to recipient vessels. Within several months, the transferred muscle becomes reinnervated by the donor nerve, eventually begins to contract, and ultimately gains independent function. Because the muscle is transferred from a distant location, and innervation comes from an extraplexal source, timing of surgery does not depend on chronicity of the injury. Function provided by the FFMT most commonly is elbow flexion but also includes elbow extension, finger and wrist extension, and grasp, even in cases of complete plexus avulsion.[28–32] It is a complex procedure that should be considered only after more simple procedures are no longer options for reconstruction.[33,34]

FFMT was originally described by Ikuta and colleagues[35] in 1979 for restoring elbow flexion in a chronic brachial plexus injury in a child. Since then, it has been indicated for use in patients who present late (>12 months) or those for whom previous attempts at restoring elbow flexion failed.[7,9,10,36] However, application of free-functioning gracilis muscles in acute (<6 months) brachial plexus injuries is being used more frequently to obtain prehension and improve elbow flexion strength.[28–30,38] Current indications for FFMT in brachial plexus injuries include when reinnervation of native musculature is not possible (ie, traumatic loss of muscle), late reconstruction (ie, >12 months), previously failed reconstruction, or for acute injuries to restore prehension.

HISTORY

Tamai and colleagues[37] performed the first microneurovascular muscle transfer in 1970 with a successfully transferred rectus femoris muscle to the forelimb in a canine and showed electrophysiologic evidence of muscle reinnervation after the transfer. The first clinical application of a muscle transfer was reported 6 years later by Shanghai Sixth People's Hospital. They reported successful transfer of the lateral portion of the pectoralis major muscle in a patient who had Volkmann's ischemic contracture.[39] In the same year, Harii and colleagues[40] reported the microneurovascular transfer of the gracilis for facial reanimation in patients with Bell's palsy. Ikuta[35] performed the

first free-functioning gracilis transfer in 1979. Since then, multiple centers have reported on the success of FFMT to restore function of the extremities and for facial reanimation.[2,28–33,40–51]

The indications for FFMT are ever-expanding and even include novel applications such as oral and anal competence.[52,53] The upper extremity, however, is unique in its importance of function in daily life and severe morbidity with loss of muscular function, and therefore much work has focused on the restoration of upper extremity function after muscle trauma or denervating injuries with FFMT.

Surgical Planning

As with tendon transfers, the FFMT should have strength and excursion similar to the muscles they are intended to replace.[42] An extraplexal nerve must be available to power the transfer, a donor artery and vein must be available to provide the necessary vasculature to the muscle. Lastly, the joints must be supple, and their motion will be restored after transfer.

The function of the muscle in its native location must be expendable and not result in significant impairment. The appropriate muscle for transfer is selected based on several parameters, including strength (force-generating capacity), excursion, neurovascular pedicle anatomy, and donor-site morbidity. The latissimus dorsi, pectoralis major, tensor fascia lata, and rectus femoris have all been used for brachial plexus reconstruction.[17,54] However, because of the anatomy of the gracilis muscle (proximal neurovascular pedicle and muscle belly, distal long tendon, long nerve pedicle length), it has become the most commonly selected muscle for transfer.[2,4,28–30,31,46,47,55,56]

Strength

The strength of the muscle is determined by its cross-sectional area, volume, and position (torque). A muscle's cross-sectional area is measured after sectioning perpendicular to its fiber direction. The volume of a muscle correlates to the cross-sectional area and provides a good measure for determination of the force-generating potential. A muscle's points of origin and insertion relative to the joint center axis of rotation determine its torque and can be affected by the way it is inset.[57]

The latissimus dorsi and gracilis muscles are poorly matched to the biceps muscle based on their cross-sectional area. Regarding strength, the rectus femoris muscle provides the best match to the biceps. However, its excursion, donor site morbidity, and less-favorable pedicle anatomy make it less desirable for transfer for elbow flexion.[31] Furthermore, the unexpectedly satisfactory results obtained with gracilis transfer, combined with its favorable anatomy, exceptional length, favorable distal tendon for transfer, and lack of donor site morbidity, have made it the preferred choice among most brachial plexus reconstructive surgeons.[2,4,28,31,35,48,55,56,58–61]

Excursion

A muscle's excursion is directly related to its fiber length and is affected by fiber orientation relative to the direction of the muscle's directional pull. Excursion of the transferred muscle should ideally be equal or exceed the normal motion at the recipient site. In general, excursion is approximately equal to 40% of resting muscle fiber length.[57] Strap muscles have fibers that run parallel to the muscle axis, whereas pennate muscles have fibers that run oblique to the directional axis. Excursion is affected by fascial constraints, bowstringing, and spanning the muscle across more than one joint.[28] Excursion requirements range from about 3 cm for wrist flexion or extension to approximately 7 cm for finger flexion. The mean resting fiber length of the gracilis muscle is 26 cm; 23 to 28 cm for the latissimus, and 8 cm for the rectus femoris.[62]

Anatomic Considerations

The quality of the distal and proximal tendons and the vascular and motor nerve anatomy determine a particular muscle's suitability for transfer. Mathes and Nahai[63] described the vascular anatomy relevant to free-functioning muscle transfer, classifying the muscles into five different types:

Type I muscles have a single vascular pedicle (ie, rectus femoris).
Type II muscles have a major vascular pedicle with minor pedicle contributions (ie, gracilis).
Type III muscles have two dominant pedicles, either of which can provide independent vasculature for the muscle (ie, rectus abdominis).
Type IV muscles have a segmental blood supply with minor pedicles that are not capable of independently providing vasculature for the muscle (ie, sartorius).
Type V muscles have a dominant pedicle in addition to a separate segmental supply, either of which may support the muscle (ie, latissimus dorsi).

All types are appropriate for transfer, except for type IV muscles because of their segmental blood supply. Motor nerve anatomy has not been similarly described for muscles but may be considered similarly. Segmental innervation, such as the intercostal innervation of the rectus abdominus muscle, prevents its use as a free-functioning muscle transfer. In the ideal muscle, a single motor nerve

is in a proximal location on inset. Lastly, the proximal and distal tendons should be strong and of sufficient length to provide strong and stable fixation in their new position.

Patient Considerations

Not all patients are appropriate candidates for such a complex procedure. Patients must understand the inherent risks, including flap loss, and the expected outcomes. They must be prepared to undergo a major operation with hospitalization and extensive rehabilitation, with the small but real possibility of little to no improvement. Although this process can be laborious and time-consuming for the surgical team, it is an essential component of the preoperative visit.

Proximal stability (shoulder) and supple joints should be assured before elbow flexion is restored. If full passive range of motion is lacking, therapy or capsular release of the elbow are indicated to restore motion before FFMT. Although shoulder stability is not a prerequisite for FFMT for elbow flexion, it should be discussed with the patient. If the shoulder is subluxed, an FFMT that is anchored to the clavicle/acromion will initially use some of its force to reduce the subluxed shoulder and thus have diminished elbow flexion strength.

The native bed for the transferred muscle must be assessed for adequacy of skin coverage and scarring. The bed must allow for muscle and tendon gliding and ideally rest in a bed free of adherent scar. However, this may not always be possible in cases of brachial plexus injury. If the skin is significantly scarred, coverage of the muscle transfer may be an issue, particularly the distal end of the muscle and tendon. Transferring the muscle with a skin paddle may help; however, this is reliable only proximally for the gracilis myocutaneous flap.[14] If muscle coverage of exposed structures or hardware is necessary, using the muscle transfer for this "dual purpose" is probably not a good idea given the inevitable scarring and immobility that will result.

An expendable motor nerve must be present near the transferred muscle's neurovascular pedicle. In patients who have brachial plexus injury, the motor nerve is usually supplied from an extraplexal source. The most commonly selected donor nerves include the spinal accessory and intercostal nerves. The function of the spinal accessory nerve can be assessed clinically through evaluating trapezius muscle function (shoulder shrug). Its strength should be compared with the opposite side, and EMG should confirm functional innervation before the spinal accessory nerve is transferred.

Trauma sufficient to cause brachial plexus injury may also cause rib fractures and concomitant injury to the intercostal nerves. Chest radiograph, EMG, and direct stimulation during the operation are the usual methods to infer or assess function of the intercostal nerves. At surgery, the motor nerve to power the muscle transfer must be confirmed as functional before harvesting the flap. Additionally, enough length is required to provide a direct coaptation of the donor nerve to the obturator motor branch of the gracilis. Interposition nerve grafts are highly discouraged and are not used for FFMT in the authors' practice.

Local vasculature must be assessed. In cases of brachial plexus injury, especially when the first rib has been fractured, the axillary and subclavian vessels are susceptible to injury.[64,65] In the authors' experience, a normal peripheral pulse examination does not preclude vascular injury, especially in the major branches. Therefore, they formally evaluate the vasculature with magnetic resonance angiography, CT angiography, or conventional angiography to evaluate the thoracoacromial trunk, which is their preferred arterial source. The vessels may show areas of thickening, suggesting vascular trauma or that the major terminal branches, such as the thoracoacromial trunk, may not be intact. In these cases, one must be prepared to explore alternative options for the vascular anastomoses, including vein graft, arteriovenous loop preparation, and end-to-side anastomosis into the axillary artery.

In patients who have pan-plexal injury, full functional recovery is not currently achievable. The generally accepted priorities in upper extremity reconstruction[15,33] include elbow flexion as the highest priority, followed by shoulder stability/motion, grasp function, hand sensibility, and intrinsic function. Therefore, most FFMTs for brachial plexus injury are performed for elbow flexion. The muscle can be inserted in a manner that also provides some finger flexion[28] or a second muscle transfer can be performed to provide prehension.[29,30,32,66] Although some authors have used the gracilis as an FFMT to restore deltoid function, it is primarily used in traumatic loss of deltoid muscle or secondary to tumor reconstruction, in which the suprascapular nerve remains intact.[34] In the authors' experience, modifications of insertion and origin sites can allow the FFMT to also act as an elbow extender.

TECHNIQUE FOR FREE-FUNCTIONING MUSCLE TRANSFER

The surgical transfer of a FFMT is a lengthy procedure, and careful preparation of the patient is important. Adequate padding and positioning to protect bony prominences and provide adequate exposure of donor and recipient sites are critical. Maintaining body core temperature facilitates peripheral tissue perfusion. The use of fluid warmers, control of ambient temperature, coverage of exposed skin, and use of warming devices should begin as the patient enters the operating room and continue into the recovery period.

Initial dissection is performed at the recipient site, generally before any dissection of the probable donor muscle is performed. If the soft tissues and skin are in good condition, initial assessment of the recipient site should determine that a mechanically sound site exists to which the muscle origin may be attached, and ensure a distal insertion will also be possible, generally to the tendon of insertion, providing the desired motion.

Verifying that recipient site vessels and motor nerves are undamaged is the final major step before proceeding to FFMT (**Fig. 1**). At the authors' institution, the thoracoacromial trunk is preferred for vascular anastomoses when using the FFMT for elbow flexion or combined elbow flexion and wrist/finger extension, as described by Doi et al.[29] The thoracodorsal vessels are used when the free muscle is transferred for finger flexion. The spinal accessory or intercostal motor nerves provide acceptable nerve function, and the phrenic nerve remains an alternative choice when no plexal nerves are available, as is usually the case. Staged reconstruction with contralateral C7 also has been described, but only preliminary results have been reported.[67] In these cases, a contralateral C7 is prolonged with nerve grafts and the distal end of the nerve is banked until a Tinel's sign reaches the distal end. An FFMT is then performed.

Once recipient nerve and vessels are dissected and their adequacy verified, muscle harvest begins. Muscle ischemic time is important to minimize (<60 minutes) through careful preparation of the recipient site vessels, including preventing or correcting vasospasm with topical vasodilators and verifying adequate outflow before the muscle blood supply is interrupted. The microscope and vascular clamps should be in place, and the muscle origin and insertion points exposed and prepared for immediate repair before muscle transfer.

Dissection of the recipient nerve should maximize its length, and the probable required length of donor motor nerve should be determined to ensure that no interposition graft would be necessary (see **Fig. 1**). At the donor site, every attempt is made to maximize vessel and nerve length, because extra tissue is easily excised but

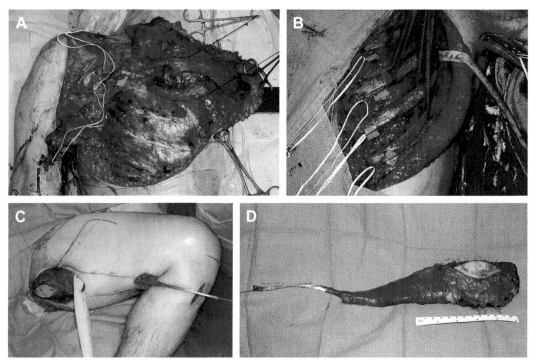

Fig.1. The recipient site is prepared (*A*) with isolation of the thoracoacromial artery, cephalic vein, and intercostal motor nerves (*B*). The motor nerve and vascular pedicle of the gracilis are identified in the interval between the adductor longus and gracilis muscle (not shown). The gracilis is freed from its remaining soft tissue attachments and divided distally (*C*) and proximally before division of the vascular pedicle and transfer (*D*).

inadequate vessel or nerve cannot be easily corrected. The authors also prefer to harvest all muscles with a skin paddle for postoperative monitoring purposes.

GRACILIS HARVEST

The gracilis is a superficial muscle that lies on the medial aspect of the thigh. A branch of the obturator nerve enters the muscle obliquely just cephalad to the major vascular pedicle, at a point 6 to 12 cm from its origin. The dominant arterial supply is provided by a branch from the profunda femoris artery 8 to 12 cm from the muscular origin and is approximately 4 to 6 cm long. The vascular pedicle is dissected between the adductor magnus (posteriorly) and adductor longus (anteriorly).

Harvest of the gracilis for FFMT begins with identifying the distal tendon at the tibial insertion (see **Fig. 1**). A longitudinal incision is made over the pes anserine, the sartorius fascia is elevated, and the pes anserine identified. The superior tendon is that of the gracilis muscle, whereas the inferior tendon is that of the semitendinosis muscle. The gracilis tendon is isolated, keeping its distal attachment. A distal medial thigh incision is

made to identify the myotendinous junction of the gracilis. All attachments to the gracilis tendon are freed at this level. Through distal and outward retraction, the muscle is placed on tension and can be easily palpated, and the outline of the underlying muscle is drawn on the skin along its length.

The gracilis is routinely transferred with a proximal skin paddle for postoperative flap monitoring.[34,41,68] A handheld Doppler is used to identify myocutaneous perforators in the proximal one third of the muscle flap. An elliptic incision is designed to incorporate these perforators in the skin paddle. The anterior incision is made and dissection is directed toward the adductor longus muscle. The fascia over the adductor longus muscle is divided and retracted away from the gracilis muscle. In the interval between the adductor longus and gracilis, and the vascular pedicle and motor nerve are identified. Vascular perforators to the adductor longus muscle are identified and ligated or cauterized as the pedicle is dissected to the profunda femoris vessels. The posterior incision is made and dissection is carried to the adductor magnus muscle. The fascia is opened, leaving a fascial sling around the gracilis muscle, incorporating the fascia from the adductor magnus and adductor longus muscles. The motor branch to the gracilis from the obturator nerve is dissected as far proximal as possible. Maximal dissection of the obturator nerve can obtain 10 cm or more of length. Preserving nerve length is important to avoid the need for nerve grafts. The nerve can always be trimmed at inset to minimize the distance required for nerve regeneration and reinnervation of the FFMT.

Before harvest and division of the muscle's proximal and distal attachments, the resting tension can be marked with sutures placed at 5-cm intervals. Although the authors no longer routinely perform this step, it can facilitate appropriate tensioning of the muscle. The distal tendon is then divided and passed to the proximal wound, and gently pulled through to the proximal thigh wound. The secondary pedicle is identified and ligated. The fascial sling around the gracilis is preserved by complete release of the fascia from the adductor magnus and adductor longus muscles. The distal tendon is replaced in its native bed and the proximal tendon is released from the pubic ramus. When the recipient bed is fully prepared, the vascular pedicle is ligated proximally and divided. Any remaining soft tissue attachments are released and the muscle is transferred to the arm.

Once transferred, the proximal tendon is expeditiously secured to the acromion/clavicle. The authors use suture anchors preplaced in the lateral clavicle and acromion to quickly attach the gracilis for elbow flexion. The muscle is placed in a premade subcutaneous tunnel and provisionally rested in its final position, but without final tension adjustment before vascular repairs. The vascular anastomoses are typically performed to the thoracoacromial artery and cephalic vein to establish perfusion, generally within 1 hour or less of ischemia time. Meticulous neurorrhaphy is then performed to the intercostal nerves or spinal accessory nerve with epineural sutures and fibrin glue as close to the muscle as possible to minimize reinnervation time. When intercostal neurorrhaphy is performed, the arm is abducted to 90° and externally rotated to 90° degrees with the elbow extended to ensure the patient's shoulder motion will not affect the nerve repair site.

Appropriate muscle tension is important for a good result, and can most easily be based on restoration of the original muscle resting length using superficial sutures placed at measured intervals along the length of the muscle before dissection, as originally described by Manktelow[41,68] and colleagues.[42] Appropriate tenodesis effect should be noted for the desired transfer because proximal joint motion either tenses or relaxes the muscle.

The authors' preference is to have the resting tension of the gracilis result in a 30° flexion contracture at the elbow.

Single Gracilis Transfer to Restore Elbow Flexion

Transferring a single gracilis for elbow flexion, generally performed in late-presenting patients with the limited goal of elbow flexion alone, is reliable when two to three intercostal motor nerves or the spinal accessory nerve is used for motor neurotization. In cases involving intercostal neurotization, the intercostal motor nerves are exposed through either an inframammary (current practice) or a parasternal incision (previous practice and used when simultaneous pectoralis major flexorplasty is performed).[28] Subperiosteal mobilization of the third and fourth ribs exposes the intercostal muscle and avoids injury to the pleura. Blunt dissection in the cephalad portion of each intercostal muscle identifies the intercostal motor nerve, confirmed using a nerve stimulator. Intercostal nerves 3 and 4 were primarily used as donor nerves based on their proximity to the harvested gracilis neurovascular pedicle. The intercostal nerves were dissected distally to the point at which muscle contraction ceased (generally near the costochondral cartilage junction) and proximally to the anterior axillary line.

When the spinal accessory nerve is used, it is identified on the deep anterior surface of the trapezius muscle, also confirmed with a nerve stimulator. The most proximal motor branch to the trapezius is identified and maintained to preserve muscle function. The remainder of the motor branch is mobilized for neurotization, sacrificing other trapezial motor branches as necessary to facilitate mobilization and nerve transposition beneath the clavicle. Arterial perfusion is achieved through connecting the brachial artery, thoracoacromial trunk, axillary artery, or lateral pectoral artery with their venae comitantes or the cephalic vein used for venous anastomosis.

In patients seen within 3 to 6 months of injury, the brachial plexus is explored and root avulsion confirmed through intraoperative somatosensory evoked potentials before selecting FFMT. In long-standing paralysis (>9 months after injury), no plexus exploration is undertaken. The gracilis muscle is dissected and the recipient site prepared to receive the transfer before its vascular pedicle is divided.

Once freed from the leg, it is brought immediately to the arm and positioned within the recipient site, in most cases for elbow flexion. In these cases, it is desirable to position the gracilis muscle as close to the donor motor nerve as possible to minimize reinnervation time and avoid use of an intercalated nerve graft. The gracilis is then sutured into place as previously described. Dissecting the spinal accessory nerve as distally as possible generally permits its passage beneath the clavicle and places it near the base of the gracilis neurovascular pedicle. The muscle is tunneled subcutaneously to a separated antecubital incision. End-to-end or end-to-side arterial connections are acceptable. When the thoracoacromial trunk is used (the preference at the authors' institution), direct end-to-end arterial repair is most appropriate, followed by venous anastomosis to the cephalic vein. The distal tendon is secured to the biceps tendon using a Pulvertaft weave after the vascular anastomoses and neurorrhaphy are complete (**Fig. 2**). Tensioning of the transferred muscle is performed with the arm held in 30° of flexion with the muscle at its normal resting length.

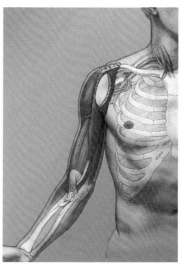

Fig. 2. FFMT (gracilis) for elbow flexion. The gracilis is secured to the acromion and clavicle proximally. Also shown are the vascular anastomoses to the thoracoacromial trunk, neurorrhaphy to the spinal accessory nerve, skin paddle, and distal tenodesis to the biceps tendon.

Double Gracilis Transfer to Restore Hand Function

Although Doi[43] originally described the double FFMT. He and others at his institution[28] have performed a transfer using a slightly modified technique. The technique for reconstructing the upper extremity after complete brachial plexus avulsion consists of two surgical procedures, each using a gracilis muscle transfer. The first stage consists of surgical exploration of the brachial plexus with somatosensory evoked potential monitoring. Currently, shoulder motor reconstruction is routinely performed, either using an available C5 nerve root, phrenic nerve, or contralateral hemi-C7 transfer.[13] The first gracilis transfer restores elbow flexion and finger or wrist extension. The gracilis is secured to the clavicle proximally as previously described. The distal tendon is tunneled beneath the mobile wad just proximal to the elbow and sutured to the extensor carpi radialis brevis tendon in the proximal forearm. Tensioning of the muscle transfer is such that full elbow flexion is permitted with a 30° flexion contracture and simultaneous passive finger or wrist extension, but allowing full wrist flexion with the elbow flexed. The first gracilis transfer is neurotized to the spinal accessory nerve, and the vascular pedicle is anastomosed to the thoracoacromial trunk (**Fig. 3**).

The second gracilis transfer restores finger flexion (**Fig. 4**). Proximally, the gracilis is secured to the second rib through multiple drill hoes. Distally, a second incision is made in the forearm and the flexor digitorum profundus and flexor pollicis longus tendons are identified and sutured together

in a position that creates key pinch and grasp with traction. The distal tendon is tunneled from the arm to the forearm beneath the pronator teres to create a pulley effect. The tendon is woven into the previously prepared flexor digitorum

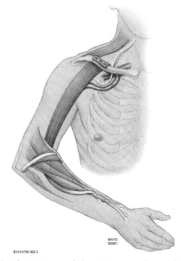

E1014709-002-0

Fig. 3. The first stage of the Doi procedure. The gracilis is secured to the clavicle proximally and tunneled deep to the brachioradialis and radial wrist extensors with the flexor carpi ulnaris pulley (**Fig. 5**). The distal gracilis tendon is secured to the radial wrist extensors using a Pulvertaft weave. (*Courtesy of* the Mayo Clinic, Rochester, MN; with permission.)

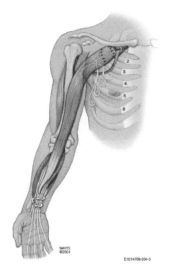

Fig. 4. FFMT for prehension, the second-stage Doi procedure. Intercostal nerve transfer is performed to power the muscle. The gracilis is secured proximally to the second and third ribs and distally to finger flexor tendons. Note a skin paddle is usually performed and the muscle is tunneled beneath the pronator teres for a pulley effect (not shown). (*Courtesy of* the Mayo Clinic, Rochester, MN; with permission.)

profundus and flexor pollicis longus tendons using a Pulvertaft weave (see **Fig. 4**). The graft is tensioned to allow fingers to extend with elbow flexion and to permit the fingers and thumb to close with elbow extension. The second gracilis transfer is neurotized by two intercostal motor nerves, and the vascular pedicle is anastomosed to the thoracodorsal artery and vein. In addition to the second gracilis transfer, the second stage of the double FFMT requires neurotization of two intercostal motor nerves to the motor branch of the triceps brachii muscle. Restoration of elbow extension allows distal joint function, provided by the free-functioning muscles crossing the elbow, through allowing its active stabilization. Without triceps function, useful grasp does not occur because elbow flexion occurs simultaneously with grasp. Finally, sensory neurotization of the lateral portion of the median nerve with sensory intercostal nerves is performed to restore protective hand sensibility.

The technique described by Doi was modified at the authors' institution.[28,30,33,35,58] In the first stage, the gracilis is secured distally to wrist extensors instead of finger extensors, which should augment finger flexion through a tenodesis effect that is not possible when the gracilis is secured to finger extensors. Because many patients develop bowstringing of the gracilis across the antecubital fossa, the flexor carpi ulnaris (FCU) has

been used to create a pulley in the proximal forearm in a secondary tune-up procedure (**Fig. 5**). Eliminating bowstringing also improves muscle excursion and wrist extension.

Postoperatively, patients are maintained in the intensive care unit (ICU) where they undergo hourly flap monitoring, including inspection of the skin paddle for color, turgor, and capillary refill time, and Doppler examination of the vascular pedicle or myocutaneous perforators. Patients are kept well hydrated, with urinary output closely monitored for signs of dehydration. Ambient room temperature is maintained at 80°F. Passive range of motion of uninvolved joints is begun immediately, as are antiedema measures. After 48 hours, patients are transferred from the ICU and progressively mobilized. Most patients are dismissed from the hospital by the fifth postoperative day.

OUTCOMES AFTER FREE-FUNCTIONING MUSCLE TRANSFER

Several authors have reported good to excellent results from transfer of a single gracilis muscle for elbow flexion.[4,28,35,47,48,58,60,61,69] In the authors' experience, 79% of patients who undergo a single gracilis muscle transfer for elbow flexion alone experienced MRC grade 4 strength or better. Using the muscle for dual purpose, as in stage I of the Doi procedure, decreases elbow flexion strength, with only 63% of patients experiencing M4 strength or greater in the authors' series.[28] Two patients in this series did not achieve any

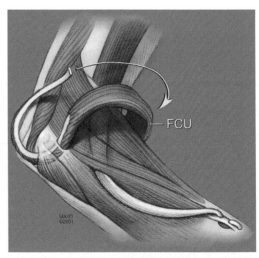

Fig. 5. Distal division of the flexor carpi ulnaris (FCU) and use as a pulley for elbow flexion and wrist extension. Note distal connection to the extensor carpi radialis brevis. (*Courtesy of* the Mayo Clinic, Rochester, MN; with permission.)

function from the transfer despite demonstrable survival.

The double free-functioning muscle transfer, reported by Doi and colleagues,[30] has similarly favorable outcomes. In their reported series 96% of patients had good to excellent elbow flexion. In addition, 65% of patients experienced more than 30° of total active finger motion (TAM) with the second transfer. In the series from the authors' institution, five of eight patients experienced some degree of finger motion, with mean TAM 30° and range 0° to 60°. Simultaneous reconstruction of elbow flexion and wrist extension compromised the strength of elbow flexion. More reliable results are achieved when transferring a single muscle for a single function. Doi and colleagues[66,70] emphasized the importance of shoulder stability and triceps (antagonist) function to optimize the results obtained with the FFMT.

SHOULDER FUNCTION

Shoulder paralysis can lead to painful subluxation of the glenohumeral joint (**Fig. 6**). Restoration of shoulder stability and balance is important for upper extremity function, can improve pain, and may make a sling unnecessary for limb control. Furthermore, shoulder stability has been shown to improve outcomes after FFMT for elbow flexion and prehension.[66]

Shoulder biomechanics are more complicated than other joints in the upper extremity. The principle joint is the glenohumeral, a ball and socket joint with multiple degrees of freedom. Secondary joints include the acromioclavicular, sternoclavicular,

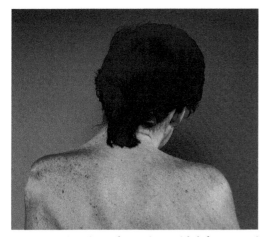

Fig. 6. Posterior view of a patient with left traumatic brachial plexus injury. Shoulder subluxation is evident and a sulcus can be appreciated between the acromion and humeral head laterally. (*Courtesy of* the Mayo Clinic, Rochester, MN; with permission.)

and scapulothoracic. These joints are together powered by a complex muscular arrangement. In general, shoulder motion reconstruction has focused on glenohumeral movement. However, scapulothoracic motion is essential for optimal shoulder function and should be considered in planning shoulder reconstruction.[59]

In his classic monograph, Saha[24] described glenohumeral function in three different groups: prime movers (deltoid, clavicular head of pectoralis major), steering group (subscapularis, supraspinatus, infraspinatus), and depressor group (sternal head of pectoralis major, latissimus dorsi, teres major, teres minor). Others have included the long and short heads of the biceps, the coracobrachialis, and the long head of the triceps as prime movers. The prime movers provide lifting power, the steering group acts to guide humeral motion and secondarily provide lifting power, and the depressor group rotates the shaft of the humerus and helps achieve full overhead elevation of the humerus. Coordinated activity of all groups is important for synchronized motion of the upper extremity.

The level of nerve injury determines the pattern of muscle paralysis about the shoulder. A preganglionic lesion involving C5 and C6 will affect all three of Saha's muscle groups, with sporadic preservation of the serratus anterior and latissimus dorsi muscles depending on the innervation patterns. The scapulothoracic stabilizers, including the rhomboids and serratus anterior muscles, are paralyzed by loss of proximal innervation by the dorsal scapular and long thoracic nerves, respectively. The rotator cuff muscles, including the supraspinatus (suprascapular nerve), infraspinatus (suprascapular nerve), subscapularis (upper, lower subscapular nerves), and teres minor (axillary nerve) are all paralyzed. However, the subscapularis and teres major muscles retain some function through their innervation from the C7 contribution through the lower subscapular nerve, and the pectoralis major muscle retains function through its C8/T1 contributions by way of the medial pectoral nerve. Both muscles act as internal rotators of the humerus and their unopposed function can lead to adduction and internal rotation contractures. The deltoid, through loss of its axillary nerve innervation, is likewise paralyzed. A postganglionic upper trunk lesion will spare the rhomboids and serratus anterior muscles, and therefore stabilization of the scapula will be preserved. Upper trunk injury distal to the suprascapular nerve will preserve innervation to the supraspinatus and infraspinatus muscles and result in weak preservation of shoulder abduction and external rotation. Loss of axillary nerve innervation of the deltoid and teres minor will prevent strong shoulder abduction and external rotation, respectively.

When nerve reconstruction with neurolysis, nerve grafting, or nerve transfer fails, secondary reconstruction is indicated. Secondary reconstruction includes release of soft tissue contracture, tendon transfers, and occasionally derotational osteotomies of the humerus and arthrodesis.

The priorities pertaining to shoulder reconstruction in functional restoration of the upper extremity are pain relief (from painful subluxation), stability, and restoration of abduction/forward flexion and external rotation. The complex biomechanics of the shoulder are often prohibitive of complete functional restoration. However, if the shoulder is stable and painless, this can be a great benefit to patients and enable functional use of the limb. The motions of the shoulder required for functional activities include abduction and external rotation. These motions aid tremendously in positioning the arm, forearm, and hand in space to perform necessary functions.

Tendon transfers about the shoulder must follow the same tenets as those for restoration of hand function, including (1) a supple joint with normal range of motion, (2) adequate strength of donor muscle, (3) expendable function of donor muscle, (4) adequate excursion and amplitude of donor muscle to provide the intended function, (5) single function of donor muscle, (6) straight line of pull of the donor muscle, and (7) synergistic function of the donor muscle to its new purpose.

Abduction and Forward Flexion

Restoration of shoulder abduction and forward flexion from loss of supraspinatus and deltoid function can be restored with trapezius transfer. This procedure was first described by Mayer[71] in 1927 and subsequently modified by Bateman[22] and Saha.[24] It involves transfer of the trapezius with its acromial insertion to the humeral shaft distal to the greater tuberosity with screw (and washer) fixation. The shoulder should be abducted 90° for distal fixation and improve the power of the lever arm.[24]

A further modification by Ruhmann and colleagues[23] involved medial advancement of the deltoid over the transferred trapezius with repair under maximal tension. This modification resulted in improved shoulder stability in their study, but only modestly improved abduction and forward flexion. In Saha's[24] original report, the trapezius was used to replace the deltoid as the primary mover, and the levator scapulae and sternocleidomastoid were used to replace the supraspinatus

as the vertical steerer. Transfer of the sternocleidomastoid and supraspinatus are rarely practiced today because of the lack of added function over trapezius transfer alone. The authors' current technique is illustrated in **Fig. 7**.

External Rotation and Internal Rotation Contracture

A problem primarily in incomplete brachial plexus injuries, internal rotation and adduction contractures occur because of the unopposed action of the subscapularis, teres major, and pectoralis major muscles. To restore function, the shoulder joint must be supple, with full range of motion. These contractures are primarily seen in late obstetric birth palsy, and are uncommon in adult patients. However, if a contracture exists, it must be addressed before muscular reconstruction.

Avoiding a contracture with passive range of motion exercises and frequent removal of the sling (which holds the arm in adduction and internal rotation) is ideal. Involving a therapist may be indicated to guide therapy. Releasing the subscapularis muscle is performed using an anterior approach and the origin of the muscle is detached from the medial border of the scapula in the manner described by Gilbert and colleagues.[72–74] The result is significant improvement in external rotation, but recurrent deformity can occur in most patients.[72] Other experts recommend releasing the pectoralis major muscle and simultaneously transferring the latissimus dorsi and teres major muscles, with satisfactory results.[75,76]

An arthroscopic approach, with release of the tendinous insertion of the subscapularis, was recently described.[77] Tendon transfer for external rotation, however, is contraindicated unless patients have restored abduction power through tendon transfer or deltoid function, because shoulder abduction must be intact for function of the external rotation tendon transfers.[78]

Derotational humeral osteotomy represents another way to place the hand and forearm in a more functional position.[79,80] This procedure involves an osteotomy above the deltoid insertion and external rotation of the distal segment at least 30°.[60] Derotational humeral osteotomy can be performed as an alternative to latissimus and teres major tendon transfer or as a salvage operation after that procedure fails.[78,80]

Arthrodesis

Shoulder arthrodesis is reserved for patients who have persistent pain and subluxation for whom previous attempts at functional reconstruction failed, although it results in a stable shoulder with

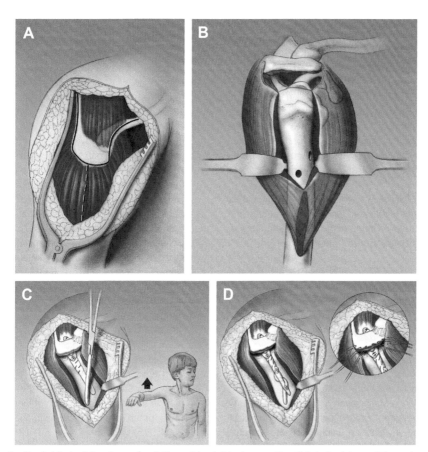

Fig. 7. A longitudinal skin incision is made at the midpoint between the distal clavicle and the spine of the scapula, and is carried down over the midportion of the lateral head of the deltoid, continuing distally in line with the shaft of the humerus. The trapezius is then elevated along its bony insertion on the spine of the scapula, the acromion, and the distal portion of the clavicle (*A*). The lateral head of the deltoid is split in line with its fibers distally, exposing the proximal humerus. The trapezius is freed of its insertion entirely and reflected proximally. The subacromial space is identified and cleared of any adhesions in preparation for the rerouting of the trapezius. Drill holes are placed in the humerus just distal to the deltoid insertion in a transverse orientation (*B*). Tensor fascia lata is used as a tendon graft. It is secured to the trapezius tendon using a Pulvertaft weave (*C*) and tunneled through the humeral drill holes. The shoulder is abducted 90° degrees and the tendon graft is pulled taut and secured back to itself using a Pulvertaft weave. The deltoid is repaired to the acromion using the previously placed sutures (*D*).

significant pain relief. The optimal position is debated in the literature;[25–27] however, it should allow for hand-to-face action with elbow flexion, typically 10° to 15° forward flexion, 10° to 15° abduction, and 45° external rotation.[81]

FUTURE

Late reconstruction of the delayed or failed primary surgery of the brachial plexus is a challenging problem for surgeons and patients. This problematic area may be addressed through improved surgical techniques; multidisciplinary approaches involving orthopaedic, plastic and reconstructive, neurosurgical, and rehabilitation colleagues; improved understanding of the basic science of

nerve reconstruction; and novel approaches to late reconstruction. Novel combinations of muscle and tendon transfers are being evaluated at the authors' center and others to address the challenges.

REFERENCES

1. Allieu Y, Cenac P. Neurotization via the spinal accessory nerve in complete paralysis due to multiple avulsion injuries of the brachial plexus. Clin Orthop 1988;(237):67–74.
2. Chuang DC. Neurotization procedures for brachial plexus injuries. Hand Clin 1995;11(4):633–45.

3. Chuang DC, Lee GW, Hashem F, et al. Restoration of shoulder abduction by nerve transfer in avulsion brachial plexus injury: evaluation of 99 patients with various nerve transfers. Plast Reconstr Surg 1995;96:122–8.

4. Krakauer JD, Wood MB. Intercostal nerve transfer brachial plexopathy. J Hand Surg 1994;19A:829–35.

5. Leechavengvongs S, Witoonchart K, et al. Nerve transfer to biceps muscle using a part of the ulnar nerve in brachial plexus injury (upper arm type): a report of 32 cases. J Hand Surg [Am] 1998;23(4):711–6.

6. Merrell GA, Barrie KA, Katz DL, et al. Results of nerve transfer techniques for restoration of shoulder and elbow function in the context of a meta-analysis of the English literature. J Hand Surg [Am] 2001;26(2):303–14.

7. Mikami Y, Nagano A, Ochiai N, et al. Results of nerve grafting for injuries of the axillary and suprascapular nerves. J Bone Joint Surg 1997;79B:527–31.

8. Narakas A, Hentz VR. Neurotization in brachial plexus injuries: indication and results. Clin Orthop 1988;237:43–56.

9. Ruch DS, Friedman AH, Nunley JA. The restoration of elbow flexion with intercostal nerve transfers. Clin Orthop 1995;314:95–103.

10. Songcharoen P, Mahaisavariya B, Chotigavanich C. Spinal accessory neurotization for restoration of elbow flexion in avulsion injuries of the brachial plexus. J Hand Surg [Am] 1996;21(3):387–90.

11. Sunderland S. Rate of regeneration in human peripheral nerves. Arch Neurol Psychiatry 1947;58:251–95.

12. Sunderland S, Ray LJ. Denervation changes in mammalian striated muscle. J Neurol Neurosurg Psychiatry 1950;13(3):159–77.

13. Songcharoen P, Wongtrakul S, Mahaisavariya B, et al. Hemi-contralateral C7 transfer to median nerve in the treatment of root avulsion brachial plexus injury. J Hand Surg [Am] 2001;26(6):1058–64.

14. Strauch B, Han-Liang Yu. Atlas of Microvascular Surgery, Anatomy and Operative Approaches. 2006;203–11.

15. Shin AY, Spinner RJ, Steinmann P, et al. Adult traumatic brachial plexus injuries. J Am Acad Orthop Surg 2005;13(6):382–96.

16. Brooks DM, Seddon HJ. Pectoral transplantation for paralysis of the flexors of the elbow; a new technique. J Bone Joint Surg Br 1959;41-B(1):36–43.

17. Hovnanian AP. Latissimus dorsi transplantation for loss of flexion or extension at the elbow; a preliminary report on technic. Ann Surg 1956;143(4):493–9.

18. Leffert RD, Pess GM. Tendon transfers for brachial plexus injury. Hand Clin 1988;4(2):273–88.

19. Segal A, Seddon HJ, Brooks DM. Treatment of paralysis of the flexors of the elbow. J Bone Joint Surg Br 1959;41-B(1):44–50.

20. Solomons M, Cvitanich M. A one-stage shoulder arthrodesis and Brooks Seddon pectoralis major to biceps tendon transfer for upper brachial plexus injuries. J Hand Surg Eur Vol 2007;32(1):18–23.

21. Zancolli E, Mitre H. Latissimus dorsi transfer to restore elbow flexion. J Bone Joint Surg 1973;55A:1265–75.

22. Bateman J. The shoulder and environs. St. Louis (Missouri): C.V. Mosby; 1954.

23. Ruhmann O, Schmolke S, Bohnsack M, et al. Trapezius transfer in brachial plexus palsy. Correlation of the outcome with muscle power and operative technique. J Bone Joint Surg Br 2005;87(2):184–90.

24. Saha A. Surgery of the paralyzed and flail shoulder. Acta Orthop Scand Suppl 1967;97:5–90.

25. Cofield RH, Briggs BT. Glenohumeral arthrodesis. Operative and long-term functional results. J Bone Joint Surg Am 1979;61(5):668–77.

26. Richards RR, Sherman RM, Hudson AR, et al. Shoulder arthrodesis using a pelvic-reconstruction plate. A report of eleven cases. J Bone Joint Surg Am 1988;70(3):416–21.

27. Rowe CR. Re-evaluation of the position of the arm in arthrodesis of the shoulder in the adult. J Bone Joint Surg Am 1974;56(5):913–22.

28. Barrie KA, Steinmann SP, Shin AY, et al. Gracilis free muscle transfer for restoration of function after complete brachial plexus avulsion. Neurosurg Focus 2004;16(5):1–9.

29. Doi K, Kuwata N, Muramatsu K, et al. Double muscle transfer for upper extremity reconstruction following complete avulsion of the brachial plexus. Hand Clin 1999;15(4):757–67.

30. Doi K, Muramatsu K, Hattori Y, et al. Restoration of prehension with the double free muscle technique following complete avulsion of the brachial plexus. Indications and long-term results. J Bone Joint Surg 2000;82A(5):652–66.

31. Doi K, Sakai K, Kawata N, et al. Reconstruction of finger and elbow function after complete avulsion of the brachial plexus. J Hand Surg 1991;16(5):796–803.

32. Doi K, Sakai K, Kawata N, et al. Double free-muscle transfer to restore prehension following complete brachial plexus avulsion. J Hand Surg 1995;20(3):408–14.

33. Bishop AT. Functioning free-muscle transfer for brachial plexus injury. Hand Clin 2005;21(1):91–102.

34. Manktelow RT, Anastakis, Dimitri J. Free functioning muscle transfers. In: Green D, Hotchkiss R, Pederson W, et al, editors. Green's operative hand surgery. London: Churchill Livingstone; 2005. p. 1757–76.

35. Ikuta Y, Yoshioka K, Tsuge K. Free muscle graft as applied to brachial plexus injury-case report and experimental study. Annals of the Academy of Medicine, Singapore 1979;8(4):454–8.

36. Chuang DC, Yeh MC, Wei FC. Intercostal nerve transfer of the musculocutaneous nerve in avulsed brachial plexus injuries: evaluation of 66 patients. J Hand Surg 1992;17:822–8.

37. Tamai S, Komatsu S, Sakamoto H, et al. Free muscle transplants in dogs, with microsurgical neurovascular anastomoses. Plast Reconstr Surg 1970;46(3): 219–25.

38. Doi K, Hattori Y, Kuwata N, et al. Free muscle transfer can restore hand function after injuries of the lower brachial plexus. J Bone Joint Surg 1998; 80(1):117–20.

39. Free muscle transplantation by microsurgical neurovascular anastomoses. Report of a case. Chin Med J (Engl) 1976;2(1):47–50.

40. Harii K, Ohmori K, Torii S. Free gracilis muscle transplantation, with microneurovascular anastomoses for the treatment of facial paralysis. A preliminary report. Plast Reconstr Surg 1976;57(2): 133–43.

41. Manktelow RT. Functioning muscle transplantation to the upper limb. Clin Plast Surg 1984;11(1): 59–63.

42. Manktelow RT, Zuker RM, McKee NH. Functioning free muscle transplantation. J Hand Surg 1984;9A: 32–9.

43. Doi K. New reconstructive procedure for brachial plexus injury. Clin Plast Surg 1997;24(1):75–85.

44. Hentz VT, Narakas A. The results of microneurosurgical reconstruction in complete brachial plexus palsy. Assessing outcome and predicting results. Orthopedic Clinics of North America 1998;19(1): 107–14.

45. Berger A, Flory PJ, Schaller E. Muscle transfers in brachial plexus lesions. J Reconstr Microsurg 1990;6:113–6.

46. Akasaka Y, Hara T, Takahashi M. Free muscle transplantation combined with intercostal nerve crossing for reconstruction of elbow flexion and wrist extension in brachial plexus injuries. Microsurgery 1991; 12:345–51.

47. Chung DC, Carver N, Wei FC. Results of functioning free muscle transplantation for elbow flexion. J Hand Surg 1996;21(6):1071–7.

48. Baliarsing AS, Doi K, Hattori Y. Bilateral elbow flexion reconstruction with functioning free muscle transfer for obstetric brachial plexus palsy. J Hand Surg [Br] 2002;27(5):484–6.

49. Chuang DC, Mardini S, Lin SH, et al. Free proximal gracilis muscle and its skin paddle compound flap transplantation for complex facial paralysis. Plast Reconstr Surg 2004;113(1):126–32 [discussion 133–5].

50. O'Brien BM, Pederson WC, Khazanchi RK, et al. Results of management of facial palsy with microvascular free-muscle transfer. Plast Reconstr Surg 1990;86(1):12–22 [discussion 23–4].

51. Ueda K, Harii K, Yamada A. Free vascularized double muscle transplantation for the treatment of facial paralysis. Plast Reconstr Surg 1995;95(7):1288–96 [discussion 1297–8].

52. Ninkovic M, di Spilimbergo SS, Ninkovic M. Lower lip reconstruction: introduction of a new procedure using a functioning gracilis muscle free flap. Plast Reconstr Surg 2007;119(5):1472–80.

53. Pirro N, Sielezneff I, Malouf A, et al. Anal sphincter reconstruction using a transposed gracilis muscle with a pudendal nerve anastomosis: a preliminary anatomic study. Dis Colon Rectum 2005;48(11):2085–9.

54. Takami H, Takahashi S, Ando M. Latissimus dorsi transplantation to restore elbow flexion to the paralysed limb. J Hand Surg [Br] 1984;9(1):61–3.

55. Sungpet A, Suphachatwong C, Kawinwonggowit V. Transfer of one fascicle of ulnar nerve to functioning free gracilis muscle transplantation for elbow flexion. ANZ J Surg 2003;73(3):133–5.

56. Akasaka Y, Hara T, Takahashi M. Restoration of elbow flexion and wrist extension in brachial plexus paralyses by means of free muscle transplantation innervated by intercostal nerve. Annales de Chirurgie de la Main et du Membre Superieur 1990;9(5):341–50.

57. Doi K, Hattori Y, Tan SH, et al. Basic science behind functioning free muscle transplantation. Clin Plast Surg 2002;29(4):483–95, v–vi.

58. Hattori Y, Doi K, Ohi R, et al. Clinical application of intraoperative measurement of choline acetyltransferase activity during functioning free muscle transfer. J Hand Surg [Am] 2001;26(4):645–8.

59. Hentz VR, Doi K. Traumatic brachial plexus injury. Philadelphia: Elsevier Churchill Livingstone; 2005.

60. Friedman AH, Nunley JA, Goldner RD. Nerve transposition for the restoration of elbow flexion following brachial plexus avulsion injuries. J Neurosurg 1990; 72:59–64.

61. Doi K, Sakai K, Ihara K, et al. Reinnervated free muscle transplantation for extremity reconstruction. Plast Reconstr Surg 1993;91(5):872–83.

62. Krimmer H, Hahn P, Lanz U. Free gracilis muscle transplantation for hand reconstruction. Clin Orthop Relat Res 1995;(314):13–8.

63. Mathes SJ, Nahai F. Classification of the vascular anatomy of muscles: experimental and clinical correlation. Plast Reconstr Surg 1981;67(2):177–87.

64. Sturm JT, Perry JF. Brachial plexus injuries from blunt trauma–a harbinger of vascular and thoracic injury. Ann Emerg Med 1987;16(4):404–6.

65. Gupta A, Jamshidi M, Rubin JR. Traumatic first rib fracture: is angiography necessary? A review of 730 cases. Cardiovasc Surg 1997;5(1):48–53.

66. Doi K, Hattori Y, Ikeda K, et al. Significance of shoulder function in the reconstruction of prehension with double free-muscle transfer after complete paralysis of the brachial plexus. Plast Reconstr Surg 2003; 112(6):1596–603.

67. Chuang DC, Wei FC, Noordhoff S. Cross-chest C7 nerve grafting followed by free muscle transplantations for the treatment of total avulsed brachial plexus injuries: a preliminary report. Plast Reconstr Surg 1993;92(4):717–25 [discussion: 726–7].

68. Manktelow RT. Functioning muscle transplantation. Microvascular reconstruction: anatomy, applications and surgical techniques. R.T. Manktelow: Springer-Verlag; 1986. p. 151–64.

69. Favero KJ, Wood MB, Meland NB. Transfer of innervated latissimus dorsi free musculocutaneous flap for the restoration of finger flexion. J Hand Surg [Am] 1993;18:535–40.

70. Doi K, Shigetomi M, Kaneko K, et al. Significance of elbow extension in reconstruction of prehension with reinnervated free-muscle transfer following complete brachial plexus avulsion. Plast Reconstr Surg 1997;100:364–72.

71. Mayer L. Transplantation of the trapezius for paralysis of the abductors of the arm. Journal of Bone and Joint Surgery 1927;9:412–20.

72. Gilbert A, Brockman R, Carlioz H. Surgical treatment of brachial plexus birth palsy. Clin Orthop Relat Res 1991;(264):39–47.

73. Gilbert A, Razaboni R, Amar-Khodja S. Indications and results of brachial plexus surgery in obstetrical palsy. Orthop Clin North Am 1988;19(1):91–105.

74. Gilbert A, Romana C, Ayatti R. Tendon transfers for shoulder paralysis in children. Hand Clin 1988; 4(4):633–42.

75. Hoffer MM, Wickenden R, Roper B. Brachial plexus birth palsies. Results of tendon transfers to the rotator cuff. J Bone Joint Surg Am 1978; 60(5):691–5.

76. Phipps GJ, Hoffer MM. Latissimus dorsi and teres major transfer to rotator cuff for Erb's palsy. J Shoulder Elbow Surg 1995;4(2):124–9.

77. Pearl ML. Arthroscopic release of shoulder contracture secondary to birth palsy: an early report on findings and surgical technique. Arthroscopy 2003; 19(6):577–82.

78. Anderson KA, O'Dell MA, James MA. Shoulder external rotation tendon transfers for brachial plexus birth palsy. Tech Hand Up Extrem Surg 2006;10(2): 60–7.

79. Goddard NJ, Fixsen JA. Rotation osteotomy of the humerus for birth injuries of the brachial plexus. J Bone Joint Surg Br 1984;66(2):257–9.

80. Waters PM, Peljovich AE. Shoulder reconstruction in patients with chronic brachial plexus birth palsy. A case control study. Clin Orthop Relat Res 1999;(364):144–52.

81. Clare DJ, Wirth MA, Groh GI, et al. Shoulder arthrodesis. J Bone Joint Surg Am 2001;83-A(4): 593–600.

Avoiding Iatrogenic Nerve Injury in Endoscopic Carpal Tunnel Release

Thomas Kretschmer, MD, PhD, OA*, Gregor Antoniadis, MD, PhD,
Hans-Peter Richter, MD, PhD, Ralph W. König, MD, OA

KEYWORDS

- Iatrogenic • Nerve • Injury • Endoscopic
- Carpal tunnel release

With rates of beneficial outcomes quoted at 80% to more than 90%, carpal tunnel release (CTR) always has been an effective surgical procedure.[1] Considering that in the United States alone more than 460,000 carpal tunnels are released annually with direct costs of US $ 1 billion, its economic impact is sizeable.[2,3] Despite this, CTR is a major contributor to iatrogenic nerve injury.[4,5] The median is now the most frequently injured nerve (41/263, 16%) in our record of operated iatrogenic nerve injuries. Obviously, some of the necessary skills are at times underestimated or not appreciated in view of the short duration of this outpatient procedure.[6,7]

In our current patient pool of 263 iatrogenically injured nerves, we have noticed increasing rates of nerve damage caused by open and endoscopic attempts at CTR since 2000. We are not attempting to argue in favor of or against the endoscopic technique, but rather prefer to delineate some of the procedure's inherent pitfalls. A recent meta-analysis of controlled trials comparing endoscopic and open carpal tunnel decompression supported the conclusion that endoscopic release has an advantage over open decompression in terms of scar tenderness and increase in grip and pinch strength at a 3-month follow-up. With regard to symptom relief and return to work, however, the data were inconclusive.[8] In principle, two different endoscopic release techniques exist (monoportal

and biportal), with additional variations (eg, extra- and transbursal Chow technique).[2,9–17] In 2007 alone, 5 of 22 iatrogenic nerve injuries operated at our department were caused by CTR (23%). Open and endoscopic CTR have their specific inherent risks for neurovascular injury. Overall, 55% of all CTR-related iatrogenic lesions were due to an endoscopic attempt.

Based on our own experience with endoscopic CTR of 170 to 220 releases per year, and after observing the intraoperative findings at revision surgery, we attempted to identify the most critical steps for endoscopic CTR to prevent neurovascular injury.

OUR METHOD

For our own practice of endoscopic CTR, we use a monoportal system. We prefer local anesthesia, with injection at the entry port just short of the distal flexor crease. Additional local anesthetic is placed in the proximal palm within and overlying the flexor retinaculum by way of needle advancement through the already anesthetized skin portion. For this maneuver, we hyperextend the hand over a rolled towel. A bloodless field is established and maintained with a combined pneumatic exsanguination bag for the whole extremity and a blood pressure cuff device. The pressure usually needs to be maintained for 10 minutes because

Department of Neurosurgery, University of Ulm/BKH Günzburg, Ludwig-Heilmeyer-str. 2, 89312 Günzburg, Germany
* Corresponding author.
E-mail address: thomas.kretschmer@uni-ulm.de (T. Kretschmer).

Neurosurg Clin N Am 20 (2009) 65–71
doi:10.1016/j.nec.2008.07.023

neurosurgery.theclinics.com

hand preparation and draping add to the time. The critical release steps are emphasized below. After skin closure, we do not apply a splint but use gauze and a mildly compressive bandage, and encourage finger movement right away to prevent hand swelling and adhesions. However, to minimize the (low) likelihood of median nerve subluxation (higher with open CTR), patients are advised to avoid wrist excursions for 2 weeks. Patients leave the hospital after an observational period of 2 hours. Before that, the dressing is changed to rule out hematoma formation or new deficits.

ILLUSTRATIVE FINDINGS AFTER IATROGENIC INJURY

Evaluation of 10 consecutive reexplored cases that were referred to our department after endoscopic CTR elsewhere revealed substantial trauma, necessitating various microsurgical repairs. The cases accumulated within only 2 years, from January 1999 to December 2000.[18] Findings in the 10 reexplored cases of previous endoscopic CTR were as follows: In 5 cases, the median nerve was injured to an extent necessitating autograft reconstruction (**Fig. 1**). In 2 cases, nerves needed extensive external and internal neurolysis. The main median nerve trunk was affected twice, the recurrent thenar motor branch in 3 cases, a digital nerve distal to the retinaculum (n. digitalis palmaris communis) 3 times, and the sensory palmar branch to the thenar once. In 4 patients, the flexor retinaculum had not been transected and in 2 cases only incompletely so at the distal aspect. A reunited, scarred and thickened retinaculum was evident in 2 cases. Three patients reported marked, symptomatic hematomas after the primary operation.

As Birch and colleagues[19] have pointed out, the more frequent risks associated with CTR are

> Incomplete decompression of the median nerve (worsens symptoms)

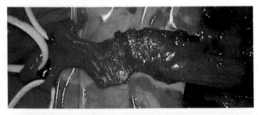

Fig. 1. Median nerve at wrist (right side) to palm level (left side) of a 59-year-old patient, after unsuccessful attempt at endoscopic CTR. The main median nerve trunk shows a near complete transection. On the left side, the common digital nerve branches are encircled with vessel loops.

> Nerve prolapse (reason why many hand surgeons are inclined to use postoperative splints)
> Injury to the main median trunk, the thenar motor branch, a palmar cutaneous branch, the sensory digital branches, or even the ulnar nerve
> Injury to the superficial arterial arc
> Painful sequelae of hematoma and fibrosis

A Sudeck's syndrome or reflex sympathetic dystrophy (now complex regional pain syndrome type I), which is usually added in the operative consent, would be an extremely rare complication of CTR.

The whole array of "pillar pain," which is a consequence of correct flexor retinaculum transection, is a subject on its own and is not discussed here.[20] However, despite its controversial nature, prolonged postoperative pain in the proximal palm can sometimes be attributed to transection of one of the tiny sensory branches that can course through the retinaculum, rather than to "pillar pain." The high initial hopes that endoscopic release would eliminate pillar pain have not been fulfilled.[21]

ANATOMIC VARIATIONS

Knowledge of the pertinent local anatomy and its variations is important for preventing disaster. Variations of the median nerve in the vicinity of the carpal tunnel will be encountered in 3% to 12% of cases.[22–26] Examples are aberrations of the median nerve itself (high bifurcation, persistent median nerve artery, calcified median nerve artery) or its motor and palmar cutaneous branches, and muscle/tendon anomalies. Among these, the more frequent ones are variations in the course of the recurrent thenar motor branch in relation to the flexor retinaculum (transligamentous 23%, subligamentous 31%, and extraligamentous 46%);[22,26] the different courses of the palmar cutaneous branch, predisposing to injury during transection of the retinaculum from below[25,27] (eg, piercing the flexor retinaculum or having connections to the ulnar nerve at the retinacular level); and various additional muscle bellies within the carpal tunnel (eg, flexor digitorum superficialis sublimis, distal belly of the flexor palmaris longus). Aberrant muscles cannot only fill the tunnel and the entry port and thus preclude insertion of an endoscope unless they are resected but, if present, they can be the main cause of median nerve compression.[28–31] The superficial palmar communications between the median and ulnar nerves deserve special consideration.[32] This connection, also referred to as "the Berrettini branch," is a frequent finding. If such a communication is at the retinacular level or in close proximity to the distal edge of the retinaculum, this branch is injury prone with any retinacular transection from underneath. A large cadaver study demonstrated the Berrettini branch in 81 of 100 cadaver hands, suggesting that this branch is a normal anatomic finding. In 28% of hands, the branch was proximal to the edge of the distal ligament and therefore prone to iatrogenic injury in one-portal and two-portal endoscopic surgery.[33] Its inadvertent transection causes sensory deficits involving the middle and ring fingers. However, in the cases we reexplored and repaired, anomalies were not the cause of injuries. In other words, serious 2injuries had been inflicted despite straightforward "normal" anatomy.

CORRELATION OF NEUROVASCULAR INJURY WITH INAPPROPRIATE DISSECTION STEPS

All parts of the distal median nerve in the hand and wrist can be found damaged. Sometimes the injuries are combined with vascular lesions to the superficial arterial arch. Partial laceration and blunt injury to the main trunk of the median nerve at a wrist or proximal palm level indicates injury with the endoscope or trocar (slotted cannula of biportal system) during insertion or dilatation. Blunt, not focally confined, extensive lesions point toward "ramming" of these instruments. Most likely, difficulties were encountered in finding the proper sagittal plane, or the instrument angle was too steep, so the nerve was hit directly with the tip of the instrument. This situation can occur if the flexor synovium between the nerve and retinaculum is not carefully separated from the nerve before insertion of the release instruments. It is essential to hyperextend the hand over a fulcrum placed underneath the wrist to ease advancement of the endoscope. Another source of damage is direct attack of the median nerve during entry port dissection, even before insertion of the instruments. In this case, the median nerve forearm sheath obviously has not been clearly identified as such and separated well enough from the median nerve. A partial or complete transection of the median nerve main trunk close to the entry port indicates a direct blade injury. This finding, in turn, implies that either the blade/trocar must have been turned around the longitudinal axis pointing downwards if the instruments were in the right axial and sagittal planes, or the instruments were passed through a plane underneath or parallel to the nerve. Damage of a palmar common digital nerve or one of its distal branches indicates that the endoscope or slotted cannula was advanced too far in the wrong plane, and beyond the retinaculum's distal edge. Not infrequently, these injuries are combined with lacerations of the superficial arterial arch. This situation is preventable if those palpable landmarks that outline the distal border of the retinaculum (hook of hamate, ridge of trapezium) are respected.[34]

Different terms are used to denote the roof of the carpal tunnel. Cobb and colleagues[35] refer to the "central portion of the flexor retinaculum" as the transverse carpal ligament, which is different from the 1989 Nomina Anatomica.[36] It is defined by its bony attachments to the pisiform bone, hook of hamate, tuberosity of the scaphoid, and ridge of the trapezium. Regardless of term preference (classic flexor retinaculum, transverse carpal ligament, central portion of the flexor retinaculum), these bony attachments delineate the roof of the anatomic carpal tunnel. They are easily palpable on a skin level (see later discussion). The first common digital nerve branches from the main median trunk at the level of the distal margin of the retinaculum. Apart from these palpable skin level landmarks, the end of the retinaculum should be visible with the camera. The retinaculum is readily identifiable because of its typical transverse fiber direction. The transverse fiber direction cannot only be seen with the endoscope (monoportal technique), but before scope insertion it can be palpated as a "rugged washboard texture," when a dilator is used. The emergence of a yellow fat pad additionally marks the distal end of the carpal tunnel, when the monoportal technique is applied. Incomplete release at the distal retinacular end indicates that the view was not good enough to recognize details, because complete transection can be nicely visualized in most instances. A dirty lens from fatty films or fluids might be the reason for a restricted, blurred view, if the scope is placed correctly within the carpal tunnel. In this case, the endoscope needs to be removed and cleaned. This requirement mainly applies to the monoportal techniques because the scope lens gliding in the slotted cannula of the biportal instrumentarium will be more protected.

CRUCIAL PROCEDURAL STEPS

For us, the best way to prevent complications with such a variety of hand morphology (eg, size of hands, thickness and rigidity of layers, subcutaneous fat at entry port, diameter of tendons and ease with which they can be shifted away from the forearm fascia) is to adhere to the same crucial steps in each case. In essence, these steps are as follows:

Identification of Landmarks on Skin Level

Their quick palpation leaves no doubt about the confines of the retinaculum, and defines the area that the endoscope should not leave (**Fig. 2**). It also allows for a good approximation of the distal end of the retinaculum.

The distal volar flexion crease crosses the proximal end of the scaphoid and pisiform bone and identifies the proximal edge of the flexor retinaculum. The pisiform bone is palpable on the far ulnar side distal to the flexor crease. Radial to it, the ulnar nerve and artery enter into the hand. The pisiform bone and hamate hook define Guyon's canal and thus the course of the ulnar nerve and artery. Consequently, the slit cannula or endoscope always has to pass on the radial side of the hamate hook, rather than blindly aiming toward a certain finger. The position of the hamate hook[37] can be variable in different hands but it is palpable. The ulnar nerve will pass on its ulnar side.

Fig. 2 illustrates where one can palpate the hook of hamate and trapezium bone on skin. These bony eminences mark the distal end of the retinaculum. Kaplan's cardinal line has been defined in various ways[38,39] but its overall clinical significance has been controversial. However, it can serve to raise the awareness of an area where the thenar motor branch will most likely be located.[40] In addition, staying proximal to Kaplan's line will definitely avoid the superficial palmar arterial arch. We trace Kaplan's line as an oblique from the apex of the interdigital fold between the thumb and index finger toward the ulnar side of the hand and the hamulus (hook of hamate).[37] The most frequent localizations of the thenar motor branch have been found within an obliquely oriented oval with vertical and horizontal diameters of 10 and 15 mm, respectively, ulnar and slightly proximal to the intersection of Kaplan's line and the middle finger radial side lines.[40] It is generally accepted to stay ulnar to the lifeline of the thumb (linea vitalis) to avoid injury to the thenar motor branch with open incisions for open carpal tunnel surgery and with the endoscopic technique.

Positioning

For us, it is essential to hyperextend the hand over a rolled towel placed under the wrist. The hyperextended hand position greatly eases the insertion, alignment, and manipulation of the instruments.[41]

Meticulous Proximal Port Dissection

Meticulous proximal port dissection enables secure identification of the forearm fascia, which can then be lifted away from the nerve to allow

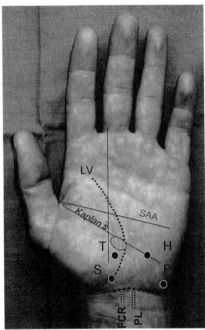

Fig. 2. Skin level landmarks for CTR. The flexor retinaculum inserts on the pisiform bone (P) on the ulnar side and the ridge of the scaphoid bone (S) on the radial side/thenar eminence. After about 2.5 cm, it will attach to the hook of hamate (H) on the ulnar side and on the trapezium (T) on the radial side. It converges from proximal to distal. The "loge de Guyon" (Guyon's canal), which contains the ulnar nerve and artery, runs between the hamate and pisiform bone. The flexor retinaculum, which is the roof of the carpal tunnel, builds the floor of the loge. A line through the hamulus and trapezium marks the distal end of the flexor retinaculum. Although Kaplan's cardinal line is inconsistently defined and cannot predict the thenar motor branch takeoff, it helps to define a corner roughly that is the distal end of an area, where this branch will be found with high likelihood (*stippled oval proximal to Kaplan's line and medial to intersection with straight elongation of radial side of middle finger*). Palmar incisions for open CTR are recommended ulnar to the hyperthenar lifeline (LV, linea vitalis), to avoid the thenar motor branch and a palmar cutaneous branch. The superficial arterial arc (SAA) is distal to Kaplan's on a line that runs from the first web space in a more horizontal direction. The distal flexor crease of the forearm (*dotted line*) marks the beginning of the flexor retinaculum. It helps incision planning for open CTR (distal to it) and endoscopic CTR (proximal to it). The courses of this subject's flexor carpi radialis (FCR) and palmaris longus tendons (PL) are marked out with dotted double contours.

for progressive dilator insertion (we use two sizes) and separation of the flexor synovium. We prefer to place this transverse incision in a skin fold slightly proximal to the distal flexor crease. It is thus easier to dislocate the flexor tendons on the radial aspect of the median nerve (flexor carpi radialis) and the more ulnar aspect (palmaris longus) away from the underlying nerve. It also allows for ample free room to navigate the instruments into the tunnel, as compared with a more distal incision, where the tendons are much more fixed in place because of the proximity of their respective insertion points.

Dissection and Dilation of Tunnel

To dissect the flexor synovium away from the median nerve, two conical dilators of progressive size are used. This procedure first creates and then widens a tunnel for the endoscopic instruments. At the same time, it supplies haptic information about the tightness of the canal. The correct plane should be reconfirmed by palpating with the smooth, broad dilator tip for the washboard texture of the retinaculum. The distal end of the retinaculum can also be felt in most instances.

Unrestrained View

It is paramount to maintain a good view, and thus to clean the optic lens whenever fatty films or liquids (local anesthetic) blur the vision. We prefer to clean the created tunnel with a rolled pointed swab to remove any fluid before insertion of the endoscope (eg, installed local anesthetic). At the same time, this procedure flattens any fat tissue remnant onto the canal wall. The endoscopic view should clearly allow identification of the retinaculum according to its color and transverse fiber orientation (**Fig. 3**A) and its distal end by emergence of a fat flap. Successful transection can be confirmed by the appearance of red muscle (**Fig. 3**B) or in very atrophied hands, subcutaneous palmar fascia (longitudinal fiber direction).

INCOMPLETE RELEASE

Two forms of incomplete release should be differentiated:

1. Failure to cut the distal portion of the retinaculum
2. Failure to transect the full thickness of the retinaculum

With the first form, the situation of the nerve will immediately be worsened because this form creates constriction and partial herniation of the nerve over the remaining edge, resulting in pronounced venous congestion and edema, which will create a vicious circle leading to more compression. With the second form, failure to transect, more space is created initially but in a triangular, cross-sectional shape. The retinaculum is left intact on the palmar surface and the full thickness will likely be reunified by fibrous proliferation exerting at least the same amount of compression as before. These patients typically complain that their symptoms never, or only initially, improved before they worsened again. On open revision, these cases logically appear as if the retinaculum has never been touched before because it was incompletely cut from the underside, leaving the surgeon's facing palmar upper side intact.

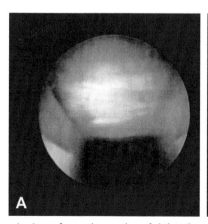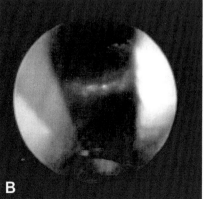

Fig. 3. Endoscopic view of carpal tunnel roof. (*A*) Before transection of the flexor retinaculum, its transverse fiber orientation can clearly be identified. (*B*) After complete flexor retinaculum transection, the overlying muscle can be seen. A view like this clearly rules out a "partial thickness" transection in the coronal plane and incomplete transection along the longitudinal axis of the endoscope.

In sharp contrast, acute new deficit and pain after CTR unequivocally delineates direct nerve injury and necessitates early open revision. Because grafting or at least an operating microscope frequently will be necessary, we prefer to do this type of reexploration under general anesthesia. Unimproved symptoms and later progression will more likely be associated with failure to transect the retinaculum, in which case a conventional reexploration with ligament transection under local anesthesia might be sufficient.

NECESSARY CONVERSION TO OPEN PROCEDURE

It is rare that a carpal tunnel will indeed be too tight to allow insertion of a slotted cannula or the combined endoscope and knife of a monoportal system. Still, every nerve surgeon applying the method will encounter situations where he or she quickly has to assess if the tunnel allows for insertion or not (eg, with a slightly different insertion angle, or another dilatation maneuver to free adhesions). It is natural that the prudent novice will thus have a higher conversion rate to open surgery. In fact, if not, the surgeon might risk complications. For the inexperienced surgeon, it is difficult to judge whether increased resistance, and maybe even sudden pain during trocar insertion, is the first sign of nerve damage or just an irritation of the nerve by the properly introduced trocar in a narrow carpal tunnel that is not fully anesthetized. It also depends on individual preferences for instillation of the local anesthetic (eg, local instillation versus plexus block). With progressive experience, conversions will actually be rare, but are still necessary at times. Our departmental conversion rate is likely between 0.5% and 2%. If the local anesthetic is injected properly, and a conventional carpal tunnel set is always in the room and thus can be opened without delay, one can easily proceed with an open procedure in the same setting. In consideration of this, the patient has given consent for this eventuality before surgery. The arm pressure cuff is usually tolerated continuously for 15 to 20 minutes without a problem. It is psychologically important to have this option readily available to avoid overriding reasonable decision making by stress and "pressure to perform" (with a patient who is awake). By hyperextension, the superficial palmar arch and the median and third common digital nerve are displaced in a dorsal and more distal direction.

SUMMARY

Endoscopic CTR is a good technique to lessen initial scar and wound pain, and to improve initial pinch and grip strength. However, it bears substantial risks for neurovascular injury. Respecting some basic anatomic and technical considerations can minimize the occurrence of adverse events. The cases of CTR-related neurovascular injuries we reexplored and repaired seemed related to inappropriate technique, rather than anatomic variations. We think that experience with median nerve exploration is an important factor to use this technique successfully.

REFERENCES

1. Badger SA, O'Donnell ME, Sherigar JM, et al. Open carpal tunnel release–still a safe and effective operation. Ulster Med J 2008;77(1):22–4.
2. Concannon MJ, Brownfield ML, Puckett CL. The incidence of recurrence after endoscopic carpal tunnel release. Plast Reconstr Surg 2000;105(5): 1662–5.
3. DeStefano F, Nordstrom DL, Vierkant RA. Long-term symptom outcomes of carpal tunnel syndrome and its treatment. J Hand Surg [Am] 1997;22(2): 200–10.
4. Kretschmer T, Antoniadis G, Borm W, et al. Iatrogenic nerve injuries. Part 1: frequency distribution, new aspects, and timing of microsurgical treatment. Chirurgia 2004;75(11):1104–12.
5. Bozentka DJ, Osterman AL. Complications of endoscopic carpal tunnel release. Hand Clin 1995;11(1): 91–5.
6. Murphy RX Jr, Jennings JF, Wukich DK. Major neurovascular complications of endoscopic carpal tunnel release. J Hand Surg [Am] 1994;19(1): 114–8.
7. Azari KK, Spiess AM, Buterbaugh GA, et al. Major nerve injuries associated with carpal tunnel release. Plast Reconstr Surg 2007;119(6):1977–8.
8. Thoma A, Veltri K, Haines T, et al. A meta-analysis of randomized controlled trials comparing endoscopic and open carpal tunnel decompression. Plast Reconstr Surg 2004;114(5):1137–46.
9. Agee JM, McCarroll HR Jr, Tortosa RD, et al. Endoscopic release of the carpal tunnel: a randomized prospective multicenter study. J Hand Surg [Am] 1992;17(6):987–95.
10. Brown RA, Gelberman RH, Seiler JG III, et al. Carpal tunnel release. A prospective, randomized assessment of open and endoscopic methods. J Bone Joint Surg Am 1993;75(9):1265–75.
11. Brown MG, Rothenberg ES, Keyser B, et al. Results of 1236 endoscopic carpal tunnel release procedures using the Brown technique. Contemp Orthop 1993;27(3):251–8.
12. Chow JC. Endoscopic release of the carpal ligament: a new technique for carpal tunnel syndrome. Arthroscopy 1989;5(1):19–24.

13. Chow JC, Hantes ME. Endoscopic carpal tunnel release: thirteen years' experience with the Chow technique. J Hand Surg [Am] 2002;27(6):1011–8.

14. Agee JM, McCarroll HR, North ER. Endoscopic carpal tunnel release using the single proximal incision technique. Hand Clin 1994;10(4):647–59.

15. Agee JM, Peimer CA, Pyrek JD, et al. Endoscopic carpal tunnel release: a prospective study of complications and surgical experience. J Hand Surg [Am] 1995;20(2):165–71 [discussion: 172].

16. Okutsu I, Ninomiya S, Takatori Y, et al. Endoscopic management of carpal tunnel syndrome. Arthroscopy 1989;5(1):11–8.

17. Janz C, Hammersen S, Brock M. Carpal tunnel: a review of endoscopic release of the transverse carpal ligament compared with open carpal tunnel release. Neurosurgery Quarterly 2001;11(1):17–25.

18. Kretschmer T, Antoniadis G, Borm W, et al. Pitfalls of endoscopic carpal tunnel release. Chirurgia 2004; 75(12):1207–9.

19. Birch R, Bonney G, Parry CW. Iatropathic injury. Surgical disorders of the peripheral nerves. Edinburgh (UK): Churchill Livingstone; 1998. p. 293–333.

20. Brooks JJ, Schiller JR, Allen SD, et al. Biomechanical and anatomical consequences of carpal tunnel release. Clin Biomech (Bristol, Avon) 2003;18(8): 685–93.

21. Ludlow KS, Merla JL, Cox JA, et al. Pillar pain as a postoperative complication of carpal tunnel release: a review of the literature. J Hand Ther 1997;10(4):277–82.

22. Lanz U. Anatomical variations of the median nerve in the carpal tunnel. J Hand Surg [Am] 1977;2(1):44–53.

23. Tountas CP, MacDonald CJ, Meyerhoff JD, et al. Carpal tunnel syndrome. A review of 507 patients. Minn Med 1983;66(8):479–82.

24. Amadio P. Anatomic variations of the median nerve within the carpal tunnel. Clin Anat 1988;1:23–31.

25. Lindley SG, Kleinert JM. Prevalence of anatomic variations encountered in elective carpal tunnel release. J Hand Surg [Am] 2003;28(5):849–55.

26. Poisel S. Ursprung und Verlauf des ramus muscularis des nervus digitalis palmaris communis I (n. medianus). Chir Praxis 1974;18:471–4.

27. Taleisnik J. The palmar cutaneous branch of the median nerve and the approach to the carpal tunnel. An anatomical study. J Bone Joint Surg Am 1973; 55(6):1212–7.

28. Schon R, Kraus E, Boller O, et al. Anomalous muscle belly of the flexor digitorum superficialis associated with carpal tunnel syndrome: case report. Neurosurgery 1992;31(5):969–70 [discussion: 970–1].

29. Brones MF, Wilgis EF. Anatomical variations of the palmaris longus, causing carpal tunnel syndrome: case reports. Plast Reconstr Surg 1978;62(5): 798–800.

30. Tountas CP, Halikman LA. An anomalous flexor digitorum sublimis muscle: a case report. Clin Orthop Relat Res 1976;(121):230–3.

31. Elias LS, Schulter-Ellis FP. Anomalous flexor superficialis indicis: two case reports and literature review. J Hand Surg [Am] 1985;10(2):296–9.

32. Ferrari GP, Gilbert A. The superficial anastomosis on the palm of the hand between the ulnar and median nerves. J Hand Surg [Br] 1991;16(5):511–4.

33. Stancic MF, Micovic V, Potocnjak M. The anatomy of the Berrettini branch: implications for carpal tunnel release. J Neurosurg 1999;91(6):1027–30.

34. Cobb TK, Knudson GA, Cooney WP. The use of topographical landmarks to improve the outcome of Agee endoscopic carpal tunnel release. Arthroscopy 1995;11(2):165–72.

35. Cobb TK, Dalley BK, Posteraro RH, et al. Anatomy of the flexor retinaculum. J Hand Surg [Am] 1993; 18(1):91–9.

36. Subcommittees I. Nomina anatomica. Subcommittees of the International Anatomical Nomenclature Committee. Edinburgh (UK): Churchill Livingstone; 1989. p. 91–9.

37. Cobb TK, Cooney WP, An KN. Clinical location of hook of hamate: a technical note for endoscopic carpal tunnel release. J Hand Surg [Am] 1994;19(3):516–8.

38. Vella JC, Hartigan BJ, Stern PJ. Kaplan's cardinal line. J Hand Surg [Am] 2006;31(6):912–8.

39. Cooney WP. Kaplan's cardinal line. J Hand Surg [Am] 2006;31(10):1697 [author reply 1697].

40. Eskandari MM, Yilmaz C, Oztuna V, et al. Topographic localization of the motor branch of the median nerve. J Hand Surg [Am] 2005;30(4):803–7.

41. Levy HJ, Soifer TB, Kleinbart FA, et al. Endoscopic carpal tunnel release: an anatomic study. Arthroscopy 1993;9(1):1–4.

Iatrogenic Nerve Injuries

Thomas Kretschmer, MD, PhD, OA*, Christian W. Heinen, MD,
Gregor Antoniadis, MD, PhD, Hans-Peter Richter, MD, PhD,
Ralph W. König, MD, OA

KEYWORDS

- Iatrogenic • Nerve • Injury • Repair • Management

It has been noted that the discretion of the protagonists generally draws a veil over the early proceedings in these cases.[1]

Injury inflicted by a treating physician has long been termed iatrogenic. In its strictest sense, however, this term is already a misnomer because it would imply "physician generating" (compare with cancerogenic). For this reason, Bonney and Birch proposed using iatropathic or iatrogenous (pathology inflicted by a physician).[1–3] Regardless of one's term preference, as long as doctors treat, patients will always be at risk for inadvertent maltreatment. Patients who undergo surgery are at risk for sustaining injury to a peripheral nerve in or outside the field.

IS IT RELEVANT TO DISCUSS THIS ENTITY SEPARATELY FROM TRAUMATIC NERVE INJURIES?

Our first evaluation of iatrogenic injuries revealed that 17.4% of the traumatic nerve injuries we operated on at our institution had been iatrogenic in nature.[4] Other nerve referral centers estimate similar rates among the traumatic injuries they operate on. Twenty-five percent of the largest series of operated sciatic nerve lesions (89/353),[5] 50% of femoral nerve lesions seen (47/94),[6] and 93% of operated accessory nerves of the same investigators were iatrogenic (103/111).[7]

Frequently, iatrogenic nerve lesions are not detected at all or not identified as such, or are approached with a mixture of therapeutic nihilism and negligence, which is why it should prove helpful to outline some of the more frequent lesions and to recapitulate the rationale for surgical intervention. Some nerves are more prone to injury than others because of their susceptibility or vicinity to the target structure. Sometimes, the particular technique applied puts the nerves at an increased risk for damage (eg, minor surgery for removal of lymph nodes at the posterior triangle of the neck, excessive use of retraction for a prolonged time (hip surgery), transaxillary approaches for the ones unfamiliar with brachial plexus pathology, or simply unawareness that the distinct pathology operated on arises from nerve [nerve sheath tumors mistaken for a "soft tissue growth"]). Although inadvertent nerve damage is often caused by poor surgical technique, some lesions might even be unavoidable with the best of preventive care.

If, as it is to be hoped, a peripheral nerve surgeon is consulted for advice, the pending questions always revolve around the need for surgical exploration and repair and the potential of recovery after such an intervention, compared with a conservative approach. For neurosurgeons, it is important to be able to give helpful advice and readily point out appropriate treatment approaches. The choice of approach will depend mainly on the lesion mechanism (direct intraoperative damage versus positional lesion or injection injury), the nerve involved, and the symptoms one is attempting to treat (pain, motor sensory, or cosmetic deficit). The intention of this article is not to give an all-inclusive overview but rather, to raise awareness of the more frequent injuries that will benefit from microsurgical intervention.

Department of Neurosurgery, University of Ulm/BKH Günzburg, Ludwig-Heilmeyer-str. 2, 89312 Günzburg, Germany
* Corresponding author.
E-mail address: thomas.kretschmer@uni-ulm.de (T. Kretschmer).

Neurosurg Clin N Am 20 (2009) 73–90
doi:10.1016/j.nec.2008.07.025
1042-3680/08/$ – see front matter © 2008 Elsevier Inc. All rights reserved.

INJURY MECHANISMS

Iatrogenic nerve injury can result from many nonoperative and operative causes: direct damage in the operative field, pressure or traction during anesthesia, injection of noxious material, needle puncture, pressure by external hemorrhage, ischemia, anticoagulation therapy, orthotics and casts, thermal injury, radiation therapy, and more.[1,8,9]

Common nonoperative causes include injection and needle injury, and external compression from orthotics and casts. Secondary sequelae of anticoagulation therapy affecting peripheral nerves are less frequent (eg, retroperitoneal hemorrhage and femoral palsy). Operative causes may be differentiated into intraoperative positioning damage and direct intraoperative damage. Direct intraoperative damage accounts for most of the lesions that nerve surgeons will have to explore microsurgically.[10,11] Of all the iatrogenic nerve lesions operated on at our institution, 94% were caused directly within the operative field.[4,12] The damage usually occurs at a distinct point of time because of a specific maneuver by the surgeon. A whole host of injury mechanisms to the nerves are possible, including being squeezed, drilled or wound up by screws; grabbed and squeezed together with the bone that needs to be repositioned; compressed by plates or retractors; torn with instruments; stretched or pinched with repositioning instruments; pierced by Kirschner wires or screws; contused by way of sudden repositioning maneuvers or simply because the forces applied were too strong (eg, clavicle repositioning with pliers for fracture plating, resulting in sudden injury and pressure on the brachial plexus); coagulated with Bovie cautery or bipolar forceps; transected because the nerves were not visualized; transected because they were not correctly identified or were mistaken for vessels; burnt; cemented or cement burned (hip arthroplasty); excised altogether with the target pathology (unrecognized nerve sheath tumors); or injured directly or indirectly by wire cerclage (eg, sciatic at buttock level, ulnar nerve at elbow level). Nerves are also inadvertently sutured and ligated (herniorrhaphy, varicose vein ligation), torn (vein stripping), or simply stretched to nonfunctionality. Sometimes, nerves cannot be visualized because the operative field is extended beyond the field of view. At the more extreme end are cases where nerves have been used as tendon grafts.[13–16] Deep hypothermia during cardiac standstill was once reported to result potentially in phrenic nerve dysfunction.[17] Open cardiac surgery (combination of sternotomy and hypothermia) has an inherent risk for brachial plexus palsy (stretch injury due to sternotomy and hypothermia).[8] Although, in retrospect, some of the reported cases of perioperative iatrogenic brachial plexus palsy might, in fact, have been due to neuralgic amyotrophy, many of the injuries described could happen despite the best of preventive measures and awareness of approach-specific risk to nerve. It is commendable if the surgeon who inflicted an injury consults a nerve surgeon for advice to initiate the appropriate treatment. Unfortunately, not only in our experience, this is still the exception.[2–4,18]

Direct and Intraoperative Damage

Procedures prone to causing nerve injury

Among the common procedures that cause nerve lesions are osteosynthesis and osteotomy, arthrodesis, lymph node biopsies at the posterior triangle of the neck, carpal tunnel release (CTR), operative varicose vein treatment, Baker cyst removal, and inguinal hernia repair. **Table 1** lists and groups causative procedures of 178 of 210 iatrogenic injuries operated on at the Neurosurgical Department of the University of Ulm from January 1990 to March 2005. In terms of procedure categories, orthopedic procedures account for most of the injuries (26%), followed by "minor surgery" (24%) and hand surgery (18%). Inguinal hernia repair (9%) and varicose vein operations (7%) contributed similar case rates to the nonoperative treatment category (7%), since hernia repair and varicose vein operations are operative treatment categories.

REGIONS WHERE NERVES ARE AT PARTICULAR RISK

Even before we observed a current drastic rise in lesions after CTR, the carpal tunnel and distal wrist (19%, or 36/191 operated iatrogenic lesions), the posterior triangle of the neck (15% or 29/191), and the knee region including the popliteal fossa (21%, or 40/191) accounted for more than half of the iatrogenic lesions (55%) we operated on until 2002.[12] In these regions, nerves lie superficial, close together, or in the immediate vicinity of the target structure. The groin remains a region at risk because of hernia repair. Surgeons treating inguinal hernias are well aware of the inherent risk for ilioinguinal or genitofemoral nerve damage. Despite awareness and preventive measures, these nerves remain at a particularly high risk because of their small caliber in conjunction with their course over or under fascia, which impedes their identification; minimally invasive procedures with mesh application might not particularly help in the recognition of these nerves.

Table 1
Case numbers of procedures that caused iatrogenic injury, grouped into categories

Category	No. of Cases	Procedures (No. of Cases)
Orthopedic procedures (26%)	55	Osteosynthesis (18) Osteotomy (7) Repair of ruptured ligament (7) Removal of plates (5) Removal of exostoses (4) Kirschner wire placement (2) Release of gastrocnemius muscle (2) Endoscopic meniscectomy (2) Myotomy (2) Open meniscectomy (1) Lengthening of Achilles tendon (1) Wire cerclage (1) Muscle fixation (1)
Minor surgery (20%)	43	Lymph node biopsy (22) Ganglion cyst removal (6) Lipoma removal (4) Hematoma evacuation (3) Abscess drainage (3) Cyst removal (2) Foreign body removal (2) Excision sebaceous cyst (1)
Hand surgery (15%)	32	Endoscopic (15) Open (6) CTR, tenolysis (5) Index finger release (3) Dupuytren release (3)
Other surgical procedures (9%)	19	Varicose vein operations (14) Removal of Baker cyst (5)
Inguinal hernia repair (8%)	16	Open (15) Endoscopic (1)
Nonsurgical treatment (6%)	13	Veni- or arteriopuncture (5) Cast application (5) Malpositioning (1) Injection injury (1) Removal of suction drain (1)
Remainder (15%)	32	Various others, not within one category
Total (100%)	210	

Depicted are 178 cases of 210 that were operated on at the Neurosurgical Department of the University of Ulm between January 1990 and March 2005.

A well-appreciated classic is injury of the common peroneal nerve at the fibular head (eg, casts, positioning). Here, the common peroneal nerve courses over and around the fibular head and neck in a superficial plane between bone and soft tissue before it branches and is therefore vulnerable to compression. The ulnar sulcus at elbow level is always of particular concern during positioning of patients.

NERVES FREQUENTLY INJURED

A full description of all nerves at risk is far beyond the scope and intention of this article. We prefer to describe a selection of nerves that will consistently have to be repaired. Our own series of iatrogenic nerve injuries operated on is regularly updated. From January 1990 to January 2008, we operated on 263 iatrogenic nerve injuries. The top 10 nerves affected have seen no major changes throughout the years. Among them are the median (41/263, 16%), spinal accessory (33/263, 13%), peroneal (30/263, 11% [19 common, 9 superficial, 2 deep]), radial (25/263, 10% [13 main branch, 6 posterior interosseous, 6 superficial sensory), genitofemoral (13/263, 5%), ilioinguinal (11/263, 4%), femoral (11/263, 4%), and ulnar (10/263, 4%). We did,

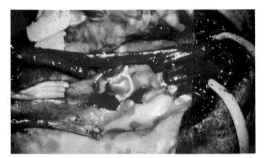

Fig. 1. Partial median nerve transection due to open CTR. Wrist level is toward the right and palm level on the left side. The nerve is depicted after neuroma resection and interfascicular dissection in preparation for placement of interpositional sural autografts of different lengths.

however, recognize an increase in referrals for median nerve injury in general and specifically after CTR. Thirty-one of the 41 median lesions were due to CTR (open: 14/31, 45%; endoscopic: 17/31, 55%), so that the median now is the most frequently injured nerve. Our rate of operated iatrogenic nerve lesions since 2000 ranges from 10 to 22 per year. In 2007 alone, of 22 operated iatrogenic nerve injuries, 5 were median lesions (23%).

Median Nerve at Wrist and Palm Level

Most of the time, this nerve is damaged from attempted CTR. The injury happens from open (**Fig. 1**) and endoscopic procedures (**Fig. 2**). For damage during endoscopic procedures, several factors can be made accountable. They are discussed separately under "Avoidance of Iatrogenic

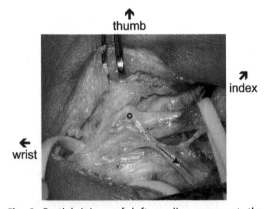

Fig. 2. Partial injury of left median nerve at the branching point of main trunk into common digital nerves due to attempted endoscopic CTR. Reexploration before dissection and microsurgical repair. Interfascicular trauma with openly displayed fascicles and scar formation can be appreciated (*star*). One fascicle group that naturally courses toward the thumb is reversed to the contralateral side (*arrow*).

Nerve Injury During Endoscopic Carpal Tunnel Release" in this issue. In open procedures, a correlation with faulty or "suboptimal skin incisions" can often be observed.[1,19] Certainly, to be secure with the more minimalized open types of CTR, expertise in regional anatomy is paramount because the surgeon also has to be able to work within tunnels to achieve complete release (eg, lifting the distal and proximal skin edges). Knowledge of skin level landmarks is of great importance for endoscopic and open release techniques. These landmarks help to project the main nerve trunk, the confines of the retinaculum, the recurrent motor branch, and the course of the ulnar nerve and superficial vascular arch on skin level before incision (see Fig. 2 in article by Kretschmer and colleagues in this issue). Because of false trajectories, severe lesions of the ulnar nerve as a result of attempted median nerve CTR are also encountered.[20] Knowledge of pertinent landmarks and variations is also important when evaluating and exploring such lesions. Passage of the recurrent motor branch through the retinaculum on the radial side is one example. Numerous variations of the median and ulnar nerve branching pattern and sensory and muscular supply have been described.[21–23] Examples include overlap of sensory supply from the ulnar side[23] (eg, communicans or Berrettini branch), or motor supply to the abductor pollicis brevis from the distal deep ulnar branch. Even after complete median nerve transection at wrist level, the possibility exists of maintained "median nerve function" due to anomalous innervation. In other words, complete transection can result in incomplete functional deficit because of cross-over supply from the ulnar nerve (and vice versa).[24,25] Therefore, this finding should not be mistaken for spontaneous recovery preventing an attempt of exploration and reconstruction. Various types of communications (so-called anastomoses) exist between the ulnar and median nerves. The Martin-Gruber varieties at the proximal forearm level can be found in 20% to 40%.[26–29] Median fascicles cross over to the ulnar nerve.[27] (The reverse cross-over in an ulnar-to-median direction at the forearm level is termed Marinacci anastomosis.[30–32]) At hand level, the so-called "Riche-Cannieu" anastomoses with exchange of fascicles between ulnar and median nerves (both directions possible) are less well defined.[24,25,33,34] After a median nerve injury, new symptoms occur immediately; at surgery, an acute, electric, shooting type of pain is noted to arise from the lesion distally to the supplied fingers, depending on the type of anesthesia applied (nerve block versus more superficial tissue infiltration). As a hallmark, a new deficit occurs after surgery and the symptoms occur acutely. Signs can be additional hypesthesia; more severe pain, which is changed in type and character (lancinating, shooting); additional or worsened numbness; and a new motor deficit. Acutely worsened and new symptoms should therefore raise the awareness for injury. As with other traumatic nerve injuries, a Hoffmann-Tinel's sign can be elicited when tapping on the skin overlying the nerve injury. Incomplete injury may especially present with a severe pain syndrome. Early exploration and reconstruction before development of a chronic pain syndrome is recommended. Incomplete or unsuccessful CTR should be differentiated from iatrogenic median nerve damage: in contrast to acute injury, symptoms do not change but preoperative complaints do not improve, and gradually become worse.

Spinal Accessory Nerve

Most traumatic lesions to the spinal accessory nerve are iatrogenic in origin.[7,35] By far the most frequent causative procedure is lymph node biopsy; Bostrom and Dahlin[36] recently described a 3% to 10% incidence. The injury is located in the posterior triangle of the neck (trigonum colli laterale). The nerve emerges underneath the lateral border of (or sometimes through) the sternocleidomastoid muscle at a distance of 7 to 9 cm from the clavicle[37] to enter the posterior triangle of the neck, which it traverses to pass underneath the trapezius muscle that it finally innervates.[38] Within its course, the nerve frequently passes in direct vicinity to a lymph node. When a lymph node biopsy is done with a minimal skin incision centered over the node and the readily palpable node is resected without a more careful circumferential dissection, it is all too easy to damage the nerve. The accessory nerve is frequently transected (**Fig. 3**), caused by tearing, cutting, or

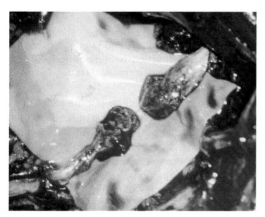

Fig. 3. Right spinal accessory nerve in the posterior triangle of the neck, found transected after lymph node biopsy.

monopolar cautery around the node's fat pad. Despite being a "motor nerve," patients often describe a sharp, electric shock–like pain during the procedure (nociceptive fibers). The true extent of the damage usually becomes evident with delay. Initial complaints of shoulder pain are misinterpreted as "wound pain" or "omarthrosis." The patients experience pain and a "pulling" sensation in the neck. Attempts to elevate and rotate the arm internally and externally ("hair-combing movement") produce progressive discomfort. Unfortunately, the correct diagnosis is often not made until the pathognomonic pattern of muscle wasting and the alteration of the scapula's position and fixation on the thorax becomes obvious. Shoulder abduction still is possible but impaired, especially above the horizontal. The shoulder girdle is wasted and a groove develops between the neck and shoulder because of the lack of the trapezius bulk. The shoulder sags down because of the lack of pull from the upper trapezius portion that inserts at the scapular spine (**Fig. 4**). At the same time, the unopposed pull of the serratus anterior muscle at the inferior angle and anterior surface of the scapula pulls the scapula down and lateral in a direction "around the thorax" (see **Fig. 4**). In addition, the upper posterior trapezial coverage of the scapula is severely diminished (see **Fig. 4**C). In conjunction, these result in a variation of scapular winging also referred to as a "swing-position" (see **Fig. 4**A); the scapula is rotated outward, away from the spine, and pulled caudally (see **Fig. 4**B). It needs to be differentiated from the "classic" scapula alata that is attributed to long thoracic nerve damage and serratus anterior palsy. Usually, the correct diagnosis is made after considerable delay. In contrast to many other nerves, the spinal accessory still seems to fare well even after delayed microsurgical reconstruction. Useful functional results can still be expected after 9 months (partly because the distance to the target muscle is short).[7,35,39] During microsurgical exploration, it is at times difficult to detect the distal stump because it has retracted considerably; in some cases, the distal stump cannot be detected at all. The value of direct muscular neurotization by use of a coapted autologous nerve graft in such cases has not been validated on a larger scale. Detection of the proximal stump and differentiation from the sensory nerves at Erb's point can be aided by direct and even transcutaneous stimulation before skin incision; the proximal stump will conduct a retrograde potential to the more proximal accessory branch supplying the sternocleidomastoid.

In cases where the functional postoperative result has been disappointing, transfer of the levator scapulae and rhomboids might be an alternative

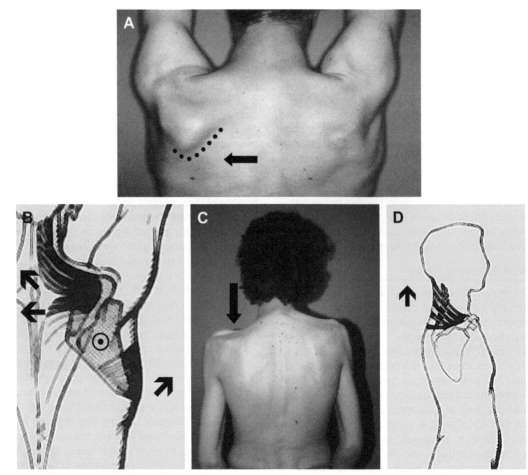

Fig. 4. Pathognomonic findings after spinal accessory nerve injury (*A, C*) in contraposition to physiologic trapezius function for fixation and movement of scapula (*B, D*). (*A*) Elevation of arms above 90° pronounces lack of trapezius covering scapula on left shoulder of this athlete. The dotted line marks the inferior angle of the scapula, which is now prominent in contrast to the right unaffected shoulder. Apart from lack of covering muscle, this is also the result of unopposed serratus anterior pull. The scapula is brought into a "swing-position" as it moves away from the spine and around the thorax in an anterolateral direction (*arrow*). (*B*) Simplified depiction of upper trapezius insertion on upper lateral aspect of scapula, and serratus anterior insertion on inferior angle and anterior scapular surface, resulting in counterclockwise turn of scapula around a central axis (☉) on synergistic contraction, enabling elevation/abduction. Right-pointing arrow indicates the direction of pull of serratus anterior muscle lateral around the thorax. Left-pointing arrow indicates the pull of trapezius medially towards the spine. Upper-left-pointing arrow indicates the pull of upper trapezius medially and upwards. (*C*) Complete atrophy of the upper trapezius portion resulted in marked groove of left shoulder girdle and sagging of shoulder (*arrow*). The scapula also moved around the thorax in an anterolateral direction (swing-position). (*D*) The main function of the upper trapezius portion is to stabilize and lift the scapula in a cranial direction (*arrow*).

(Eden-Lange procedure).[40] Results apparently are not as favorable as the ones for scapular winging because of serratus anterior loss.

Radial Nerve

The radial nerve is most susceptible to injury where it spirals around the humerus, at its proximal forearm course, and at the distal wrist, where its sensory cutaneous branch emerges underneath the brachioradialis fascia. Not only does

a dislocated humeral fracture put the radial nerve at risk, but so do subsequent open reduction and fixation. The radial nerve has been found plated to the humeral bone in all larger series (**Fig. 5**).[1,3,41] If the nerve was plated but is in discontinuity in conjunction with a grossly displaced fracture, it seems more likely that the nerve was initially torn by the fracture impact. At wrist level, Kirschner wire placement for radial fractures can pierce the superficial sensory branch. Apparently, mini incisions have been found safer than pure

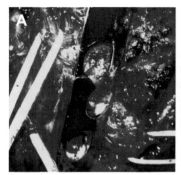
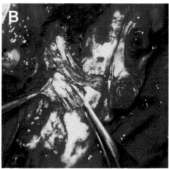
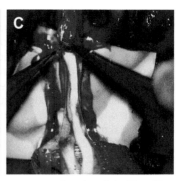

Fig. 5. Plating of radial nerve. (*A*) Plated midhumeral fracture. Radial nerve compressed under plate. Vessel loops around nerve lateral and medial to plate. (*B*) After plate removal, neuroma resection, and an interfascicular dissection prepared for graft coapted. (*C*) Sural nerve grafts coapted to proximal nerve stump with 10-0 suture.

percutaneous placement.[42] The radial nerve has an excellent prognosis for functionally useful recovery after reconstruction, with frequent full recovery of strong wrist extension after grafting, and functionally useful finger extension. In the rare case where nerve reconstruction is not an option, tendon transfers should be considered. The good motor outcome after radial nerve reconstruction is in sharp contrast to treatment results after injury to its cutaneous branch at wrist level, the superficial sensory radial nerve. Transections and partial injuries can result in painful neuropathies that are hard to treat. Among the numerous treatment approaches described, none has proved to be decisively more effective than proximal neuroma resection that allows for stump retraction underneath the brachioradialis muscle or decompression and external neurolysis of a microscopically intact nerve.[43]

Cutaneous and Digital Nerves

Damage to cutaneous and digital nerves happens far more often than comes to attention. If all cutaneous and digital nerves were grouped together, they would comprise a sizeable portion of all iatrogenic nerve injuries. When a sensory nerve is cut, dysesthesias occur and painful neuromas can develop. The symptoms can be out of proportion to the nerve's size, supplied area, and importance. Examples of frequently cut cutaneous branches prone to developing ailing symptoms are the superficial radial nerve at wrist level after Kirschner wiring of radioulnar fractures or needle stick injury (**Fig. 6**), the medial antebrachial cutaneous branch at elbow level (following ulnar nerve/cubital tunnel decompression),[44] digital nerves of the hand[45] (**Fig. 7**, after trigger finger release), the infrapatellar branch of the saphenous

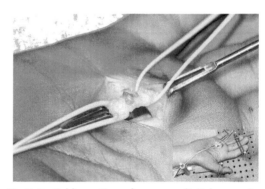

Fig. 7. Partial laceration of common digital nerve due to trigger finger release of the ring finger. Release aims at transection of the A1 flexor pulley at the metacarpal head level. Most commonly affected are the ring and middle finger and, to a lesser degree, the thumb. This patient complained of hypersensitivity and dysesthesia to the opposing sides of D IV and III and electrifying distally shooting pain on touch after such a release. The Hoffman-Tinel's sign was positive over the lesion, reproducing the pain. In this case, the previous incision at the distal palmar flexor crease was used to expose the nerve for microsurgical, split end-to-end repair.

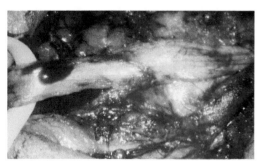

Fig. 6. Right superficial sensory radial nerve at wrist level after needle stick injury due to attempted vessel puncture, resulting in pain and paresthesia. Photograph depicts scar and neuromatous enlargement of the nerve from the midportion to the right. Interfascicular neurolysis revealed a monofascicular neuroma that was resected.

nerve at knee level after arthroscopic and open knee procedures, and various cutaneous branches at the dorsum of the foot. Frequently, no rationale exists for reconstruction because it would imply sacrifice of another sensory nerve as an autograft. The usual options are neuroma resection and burial of the proximal stump in deeper tissue layers or decompression/neurolysis. Insertion of artificial guiding tubes might be an alternative when proximal and distal stumps can be located and sensation is functionally important (eg, digital branches to inner aspect of thumb and index). The guiding matrix might at least prevent formation of yet another end-bulb neuroma because axons will be provided with a target structure. By way of nerve conduits, distances of close to 3 cm can be overcome by sprouting axons until "reconnection to the distal stump."[46–50] It is our opinion that the high material expenditure for this indication has so far prevented its broader use. Interposition of a freeze-thawed muscle graft as a guiding bridge that provides the sprouting axons with a basal lamina substitute is not commonly performed.[49]

Trunk: Inguinal Nerves

The ilioinguinal, genitofemoral, and sometimes iliohypogastric nerves are cut, coagulated, sutured, or incorporated into a mesh at open and endoscopic hernia repairs.[51] Incidences of inguinal nerve damage after open and laparoscopic hernia repair are quoted as 0.5% to 2%.[52,53] If exploration is attempted from anterior by way of the old incision, it is often difficult to identify clearly the damaged nerve within the scar and incised fascia, unless a suture or clip can be identified around the nerve. So, often, only scar tissue and possibly a contained but not visualized neuroma can be resected.[54,55] Some investigators advocate neurolysis if a nerve can be found in scar or suture but is otherwise intact. At the same time, reexploration should not leave the abdominal wall weakened with potential for recurrent herniation. Others have recommended a retroperitoneal approach to allow for identification of the affected nerve proximal to healthy tissue.[52,53] Such an approach aims at neuroma resection and deep burial of the proximal stump to treat severe neuropathic pain. The neuroma that will form again will then be protected deep in tissue. The importance of retroperitoneal placement has been pointed out for the genital branch of the genitofemoral nerve.[56] Exact preoperative diagnosis of the affected inguinal nerve is then, however, mandatory. Despite theoretic differences in innervation pattern and sophisticated, diagnostic nerve blocks,[57] it often is not

possible to clearly differentiate between genitofemoral and ilioinguinal damage. If a chronic pain syndrome has already developed ("central sensitization"), it is frequently difficult to obtain long-term relief with neuroma resection. Conservative therapy with serial infiltrations of local anesthetics and corticoids has its role before repeated surgical attempts.

Lower Extremity Nerves

Frequently, the common peroneal and the superficial and deep branch, the saphenous, its infrapatellar branch, and, less frequently, the tibial nerve are injured during orthopedic procedures and varicose vein treatment. Varicose vein surgery threatens all of the above-mentioned nerves (eg, ligation, stripping, and tearing out). The main femoral and sciatic trunk can be damaged during orthopedic procedures (**Figs. 8** and **9**) involving the femur and hip joint. Hip arthroplasty is a typical example (see **Fig. 8**).[58–61] Traction on the nerve during sustained extreme positional maneuvers, cement for artificial hip joints (thermal and mechanical damage), and the instrumentation as such, and cerclage for reinforcement of femoral fracture instrumentation are reported mechanisms. For injury to the sensory cutaneous nerves of the ankle and dorsum of the foot, Kirschner wiring, exostosectomy, and instrumentation for fracture treatment are frequent lesion mechanisms. Another procedure with high potential for peroneal and tibial nerve damage is Baker cyst removal at the popliteal fossa.

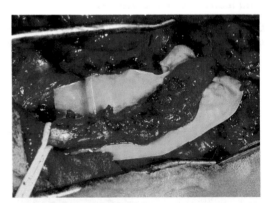

Fig. 8. Iatrogenic lesion of right sciatic nerve 6 months after cemented hip arthroplasty in a 60-year-old patient. The nerve was explored at an infrapiriformis level and found to be in partial continuity only. Cement fragments were additionally found around the nerve. Evaluation with nerve action potentials confirmed a complete injury with no conduction across the lesion, necessitating graft repair.

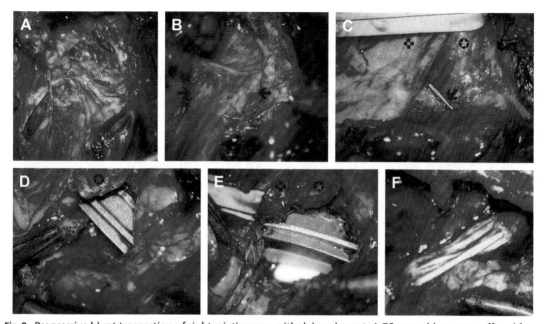

Fig. 9. Progressive blunt transection of right sciatic nerve with delayed onset. A 76-year-old woman suffered from progressive weakness of right foot dorsiflexion and L4/5 hyp- and dysesthesia, starting 5 months after implantation of a total hip endoprosthesis. Until then, she was able to drive her car. Within 2 months she developed a drop foot. Electric shock–like dysesthesias radiating from the lower buttock to the ankle severely aggravated her symptoms. At the time of presentation, she was unable to sit because of excruciating pain. Preoperative motor examination indicated the following: gluteus maximus and medius 5/5 (British Medical Research Council), biceps femoris 5/5, peronei 0/5, extensor hallucis longus/toe extensors 0/5, tibialis posterior 2/5, toe flexors 4–5/5, gastrocnemius 5/5. MRI excluded tumorous involvement; some scar could be appreciated in the area of the implant. Pelvic radiograph revealed no peculiarities. Findings at surgery: (A) A posterior approach to expose the sciatic nerve from the subgluteal fold to the notch area was chosen. Before the nerve was encountered, scar tissue was appreciable. (B) Eight centimeters caudal to the notch area, a severe adhesion of the sciatic became evident; the lateral circumference was found transected and embedded in scar tissue. Sciatic nerve and scar within arrows. (C) Further dissection revealed a metal strip abutting the nerve (*arrow*). (D) The metal edge was soon identified to be part of the acetabular joint thread, which was not completely embedded in bone. (E) The thread had completely transected the peroneal division of the sciatic (*star*), and a minor tibial portion (*cross*). (F) The neuromatous segments were resected for a split type of repair. In an attempt to prevent painful neuroma formation, the sciatic was reconstructed using eight strands of autologous sural nerve graft. A pedicled fat flap was created to cover the interspace between nerve and hip implant (hip revision was not an option). Postoperatively, the typical pain had vanished and despite her advanced age and the extensive approach, she was only on nonsteroidal anti-inflammatory drugs for a week. After days, she ambulated on crutches. She remained pain free but, as predicted, did not recover from drop foot. Adequate management of high sciatic lesions with a severe pain component in the elderly is subject to controversy.

Other Nerves

A complete list of other nerves would be extensive. Some of the more notable examples are included here. During thyroid and anterior cervical spine surgery, the right recurrent laryngeal nerve is at risk for compression from retractor blades, but most will recover spontaneously.[62,63] Transections have been reported only rarely. Wisdom tooth extraction can damage lingual and inferior alveolar nerves;[64–66] the lesion rate is five times higher under general than local anesthesia. Cranial and perimastoid incisions can damage the facial and occipital nerve branches.

FAULTY RESECTION OF BENIGN NERVE SHEATH TUMORS WITH NERVE

Every nerve surgeon comes across cases where a whole nerve segment or parts of the brachial plexus have been "eradicated" en bloc on purpose, together with a "malignant-looking tumor." Neurofibromas and schwannomas are often preoperatively not identified as such; percutaneous needle biopsies are contraindicated because they can damage the nerve and are not diagnostic enough to differentiate between benign and malignant tumors. Kehoe and colleagues[67] found that in 88 pathologically proven neurofibromas or schwannomas resected between 1959 and 1990, the correct diagnosis was only made in 7 cases, or 8%. It must be mentioned, however that most of the cases referred to in this study had been treated before more sophisticated MRI sequences were in widespread use. Benign schwannomas can be resected microsurgically without functional deficit, which also applies to the technically more demanding neurofibroma resection. Because nerve tumors are rare, the number of surgeons who have experience with this tumor entity is small. That is why, once the diagnosis is suspected, this type of surgery should be reserved for experienced nerve surgeons. An important aspect is the low predictive value of MRI in discerning malignant from benign tumors. A peripheral nerve sheath tumor with features suggesting malignancy on imaging (eg, cystic or "ancient variants") might intraoperatively turn out to be benign, if approached and dissected in the proper way. En bloc resections of benign nerve tumors are obviously contraindicated; nevertheless, they happen. Such lesions should be explored and grafted as soon as possible.[68] Lipoma resection in proximity to nerves predisposes to nerve damage when undertaken by way of minimized skin incisions without careful circumferential dissection (comparable to lymph node biopsy; see above).

Indirect Damage and Nonoperative Causes

Injection injury

The most common neural injection sites are the sciatic nerve at buttock level and the radial nerve at the lateral upper arm.[69,70] Marantic adults and children are at higher risk because of thinner soft tissue layers. Higher case rates of gluteal injection injuries have been reported from countries where serial intramuscular injections were performed (eg, chloroquine malaria prophylaxis). These injuries more frequently affect children under age 5.[71–73] In principle, intraneural injection needs to be differentiated from perineural.[2] In their experimental study, Gentili and colleagues[74,75] stressed the particular danger of intrafascicular injection. Signs of intraneural injection are instant electric shock–like pain radiating down the limb, with paresthesias, radicular burning pain, and numbing and complete or incomplete paralysis. A delayed onset of symptoms, usually in conjunction with a severe burning component, points more toward perineural deposition of an agent. Apparently, in 10% of cases, symptoms present with delay.[76] It is important to clarify if the injected agent was neurotoxic because the instant damage and the developing reactive intraneural fibrosis will be worse. Among the more commonly used intramuscular

agents, diazepam, chlorpromazine, and dexamethasone are neurotoxic. For neurotoxic agents, immediate exploration is a consideration. Two slightly different approaches to injection injuries have been described. One is an initially more observant one,[77] the other is urgent exploration in cases of instant paralysis following injection of a neurotoxic agent within the course of a main nerve.[1,2] Instant exploration and epineurotomy aim to prevent delayed internal compression by the fibrosis that inadvertently will occur because of neurotoxicity. Irrigation with saline is used in an attempt to dilute the agent. If in severe pain, Bonney[2] advised leaving a perineural catheter in place for direct analgesia with a lignocaine or bupivicaine solution. However, chances for instant referral of such a patient will be close to zero. If, theoretically, 2 to 3 days after the event, a patient were referred with injection injury, Dr. Bonney would still recommend the outlined procedure if the patient had persistent severe pain, complete paralysis within hours of injection, or progression of paralysis. Fortunately, most injection injuries will show spontaneous recovery and have no element of neurotoxicity, which is why the New Orleans group and others are more inclined most of the time to observe recovery over a 2- to 4-month period. Recovery, though, takes a long time and likely will be incomplete. In the absence of progress, grafting or split repair of the damaged segment might be necessary. Ongoing pain or severe deficits are then seen as indications for exploration. If no nerve action potential can be recorded across the injured segment intraoperatively, the lesion is resected and grafted. The best preventive measures include knowledge of pertinent anatomy and landmarks, appropriate needle length in conjunction with proper angle of injection, and accounting for the body habitus of the patient rather than injecting in a stereotyped manner.

Compressive Arterial Bleeding

At particular risk are the supra-and infraclavicular brachial plexus after attempted central line insertion, the brachial artery in the arm (attempted catheterization may cause bleeding into the fascial sheath affecting the median nerve), the ulnar artery at the elbow (blood collection in the deep forearm compartment affecting the ulnar nerve), the radial artery at the wrist (median nerve compression), the femoral artery at the groin (catheter angiography affecting the femoral nerve), and the aorta in the abdomen (bleeding down the psoas sheath affecting the lumbar plexus). If findings on physical examination are not obvious (large groin hematoma after catheter angiography and progressive pain or nerve deficits), MRI is helpful. MRI certainly is indicated to rule out potential intrapelvic or retroperitoneal hematomas, when new postoperative progressive deficits cannot be explained after orthopedic, abdominal, or vascular procedures in the vicinity of these spaces. Elderly patients under anticoagulation who undergo joint replacement are at particular risk for extraneural bleeding into a compartment causing nerve compression. A common procedure is hip arthroplasty. Intraneural hemorrhage after administration of anticoagulants like warfarin and heparin has also been described. The concurrent administration of heparin and warfarin with nonsteroidal anti-inflammatory drugs can potentiate their anticoagulative effects.[78,79] Sizeable hemorrhages resulting in symptomatic nerve compression need to be evacuated. Unfortunately, this group of patients is also at higher risk for rehemorrhage after hematoma evacuation, so placement of a drain after meticulous hemostasis has been achieved should be considered.

Tourniquet Palsy

The pathognomonic features of tourniquet palsy are that all nerves of an extremity are affected to various extents and a Hoffmann-Tinel's sign is absent. Incidences of 1 in 7000 surgeries have been quoted.[80] Several scenarios are conceivable. The chosen pressure above the patient's systolic blood pressure is too high because the surgeon does not know better (unlikely), or, more likely, the pressure is actually higher than what the manometer indicates. Safe time parameters are exceeded or the patient's body habitus has not been accounted for (eg, thin extremity). The pressure cuff can be too narrow for the extremity circumference, and multiple combinations of the above mentioned mechanisms. Recommended are cuffs of at least 14 cm width for the adult arm, and of 18 cm for the adult thigh. Application should be at the proximal part of the extremity with padding between cuff and skin. Recommended inflation pressures are 50 to 75 mm Hg above systolic for the upper limb, and 100 to 150 mm Hg above systolic for the lower limb. But recommendations vary, and 100 mm Hg above systolic is frequently used for the upper limb. A method to minimize the necessary pressure to the minimal effective pressure that maintains arterial closure has been suggested.[81] Inflation time should not substantially exceed 1.5 hours for the upper extremity, and 2 hours for the leg.[2,19] Tourniquets cannot be used over an arterial prosthesis. Some recommend releasing the cuff after 1 hour to allow for

some bleeding before reinflation. It is only prudent to adjust these guiding measures and time frames to the actual findings of body habitus and to take neuropathy-predisposing factors into account (alcoholism, diabetes, renal insufficiency, inherited disorders, and so forth). An important point is to check the accuracy of the manometer regularly.

Bonney pointed out that, in principle, any inflation of a cuff produces an ischemic nerve lesion if pressure is maintained for more than 20 minutes. However, this lesion is transient and resolves quickly when the cuff is deflated. Several investigators studied and discussed the effects of a tourniquet on muscle and nerve to find out if pressure or ischemia is the primary pathogenetic mechanism.[19,82,83] A case report of tourniquet paralysis that was meticulously followed electrophysiologically demonstrated how a combination of axonal degeneration and conduction block resolves over time.[84]

Closed Pressure or Traction During General Anesthesia

Causes are intraoperative positioning with excess pressure against body parts, where nerves lie superficially and course around or in close proximity to bone (eg, peroneal nerve at the fibular neck and ulnar nerve at the medial epicondyle), extensive pull, and constriction by inappropriately narrow straps (nerves at wrist).[85–87] At times, no distinct mistake in positioning and padding is identifiable but rather, an unfavorable combination of predisposing factors has to be accounted for,[86] including extremes of body habitus, preexisting compressive neuropathy, neuropathy in diabetics, alcoholics, dialysis patients, or hereditary neuropathy with liability to pressure palsies, and extremes of body position for a sustained amount of time (eg, lithotomy and femoral nerve lesion, lateral decubitus position and peroneal nerve injury, taping down of the shoulders resulting in brachial plexus stretch injury). All these predisposing factors are augmented by general anesthesia and use of muscle relaxants. Excessive shoulder pull (eg, taping down the shoulders with the head turned to the contralateral side) and shoulder abduction under general anesthesia are to be avoided (preferably not more than 70°); combining shoulder abduction with lateral rotation at the glenohumeral joint poses an additional risk. Yet some of these positions might be unavoidable at times (eg, for approaches that necessitate access to the inner aspect of the arm and the axilla). It is good practice to test the range of motion preoperatively with the patient awake. Bone-to-bone contact needs to be prevented by pads (eg, knees). The additional importance of hand positioning (palms up, hand supinated) when the patient is placed supine with the arms at the side to prevent compression of the ulnar nerve at elbow level has been pointed out.[77,88] The ulnar is one of the nerves most frequently affected from malpositioning. An unfavorable position is full extension of the elbow, when forearm and hand are pronated. The pressure points are in the olecranon notch or groove. Full elbow flexion is also unfavorable.[85,86]

Irradiation

The brachial plexus is the usual site of radiation neuropathy. It appears with a time lag of several years, usually after radiation for breast carcinoma or malignant neck tumors.[89] Features from history (timing or high radiation dose), physical examination (eg, skin sclerosis, telangiectasias), and electrophysiology (eg, myokymia, continuous quivering and undulation of skin surface, and spontaneous repetitive discharge of motor unit potentials) give decisive clues.[2,90] Pain and sensory symptoms are the first features, followed by motor deficit. In the beginning, symptoms might point toward the median or ulnar nerve and to a lower trunk level, and therefore they can be mistaken for carpal or cubital tunnel syndrome. It is important to include metastasis in the differential diagnosis and to obtain an MRI (or fluordeoxyglucose–positron emission tomography). The plexus elements and the surrounding soft tissue, including muscle and vascular tissue, undergo progressive sclerosis. Consequently, the nerve not only develops a diffuse intrinsic lesion but also is entrapped in scar. The role of surgery is limited to microsurgical decompression by division of the epineurium and overlying sclerotic tissue. Some investigators with considerable experience also advocate transfer of muscle or omentum to attempt revascularization. Surgery mainly aims at pain reduction and slowing of progression. Graft reconstruction is unsuccessful.

Differential Diagnosis Brachial Plexitis

Brachial plexitis, or neuralgic amyotrophy, is known under the eponym Parsonage-Turner syndrome[91–93] and thought to be inflammatory or immune-mediated in nature. It occurs after physical stress and exertion. The underlying pathomechanism still is unrevealed. It also has been diagnosed perioperatively.[94] In contrast to iatrogenic injury to the brachial plexus, its onset is delayed. The time course, intense initial shoulder girdle pain, and the subsequent and delayed onset of shoulder and limb weakness discern it from the more focal traumatic lesions to the brachial plexus. The

syndrome affects several peripheral nerve distributions in a patchy pattern that could not possibly stem from a focal cord to nerve origin (suprascapular, radial, axillary, long thoracic). To complicate matters, cases of single nerve, and bilateral plexus affection, have been described.[91]

MANAGEMENT PRINCIPLES

For treatment of iatrogenic nerve lesions, the same principles apply as for any other traumatic nerve injury. Attempts at minimizing time delay are most important for the functional prognosis of reconstructed nerves. However, as discussed, injection injuries, positioning injuries, and radiogenic neuropathy are approached differently.

Delayed Referral

Rarely, patients will be referred from the primary surgeon. Only one third of our patients could be operated on within an appropriate time interval of 6 months after the injury. Other groups report similar experiences. Frequently, patients are referred through a neurologic colleague who has been consulted on the patient's own initiative because of sustained sensorimotor deficits or painful sequelae.

Prognostic Factors Nonconditional to Surgeon

These factors are given by the type, mechanism, and level of the lesion, nerves affected, concomitant injuries, and patient age, and as such, are not conditional to the treating surgeon. Isolated, focal nerve injuries without concomitant severe arterial or bony component in younger patients generally will fare better, as do radial and spinal accessory lesions if compared with peroneal nerve injuries.[95]

Prognostic Factors Conditional to Surgeon

Other factors, however, are conditional to the treating surgeon, namely, judgment, timing of repair, and technique used. A treatment algorithm relating to injury type, with timing and repair technique, is given in **Fig. 10**. Timing of reconstructive surgery is a crucial factor for functional, useful recovery.[96,97] In general, functional outcome is adversely affected if more than 6 months have passed between injury and repair.[98–102] Repair should be attempted as early as possible, when the lesion has been judged to have insufficient potential for useful spontaneous recovery. Progressive neuronal death, ischemia, and fibrous proliferation are important limiting factors for useful recovery.[103] Experimental evidence exists for progressive neuronal death to occur after a critical

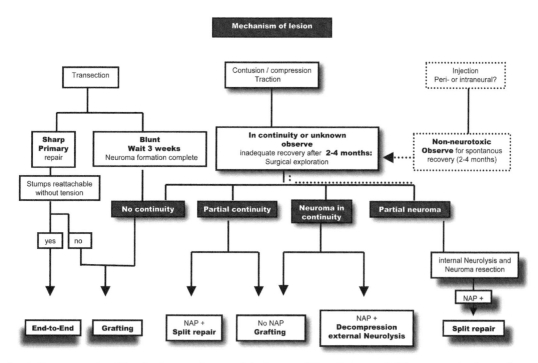

Fig. 10. Treatment algorithm for iatrogenic nerve injuries, specifying timing and different repairs depending on injury type. NAP, nerve action potential.

time window has passed. Sensory and motor neurons appear to differ in the onset of such cell loss. Evidence also indicates that early nerve repairs can stop this process of neuron loss.[104] It seems that early repair improves the reconstructed nerve's regenerative capacity. In summary, the efficacy of axonal regeneration is significantly affected by the amount of cell loss already present at the time of repair.[105–108] As far as technique is concerned, microsurgical principles apply and, as such, microinstruments, magnification devices, and proper illumination are mandatory for attempts at repair and neurolysis.

Appropriate Treatment

For those who inflicted a severe injury, we recommend contacting an experienced nerve surgeon. The first step is to evaluate the lesion mechanism. The most frequent intraoperative direct causes are transection, stretch, contusion, compression, and combinations thereof. Furthermore, the continuity of the lesion needs to be evaluated, and an attempt at grading the degree of damage helps to judge the potential for spontaneous recovery. Good electrophysiologic examinations can be a helpful adjunct. Despite the accentuated fragmentation of the lesion types outlined below, one should be aware that an affected nerve segment could show a spectrum of lesion degrees. For

instance, a partial laceration with neuromatous change of the flanking fascicles can exhibit only neurapractic changes at the marginal fascicles. Injection and thermal injuries will most likely be observed first (see earlier discussion and **Fig. 10**).

Sharp Transection

After sharp transection, immediate primary end-to-end suture is indicated. Nevertheless, instant retraction of the nerve ends might sometimes necessitate an interpositional graft or a transpositional maneuver to gain nerve length. Only the inflicting surgeon can judge if the nerve is sharply transected. However, straightforward cases like these are rare in clinical practice.

Blunt Transection

A waiting interval of three weeks is recommended if the transection is due to pull and tear (eg, stretch with tear, or drilled and wound-up nerve), and as such has a blunt element with contused margins, and if such a mechanism cannot be ruled out. The interval allows for complete formation of the stump neuromas along the longitudinal axis.[96] Then, an "early secondary repair" will be performed. The idea is to prevent coaptation of two putatively healthy-looking stumps that have no potential for recovery. The trauma might have had a far more proximal impact than could possibly be appreciated with exploration at the time of injury. In other words, it would not be clear how far back the stumps needed to be resected to meet healthy fascicular structure that does not transform into neuroma. Such a neuromatous formation would hinder successful outgrowth of axons because of its fibrous tissue barrier.

At repair, nerve stumps are cut back to healthy-looking fascicular structure, and the resulting gap is bridged with interpositional grafts. Indicators of "healthy" fascicular structure are a moist, glossy-looking surface with protruding fascicles, and lack of scar tissue; if in doubt, a frozen section can help.

Mechanism Unknown or Lesion in Continuity

Most nerve injuries will only be detected in the postoperative course because of the inflicted symptoms of pain and sensorimotor deficits. As a rule, the signs and symptoms will occur directly after surgery. For an extremely rare exception, we refer to **Fig. 9**. Unless the inflicting surgeon knows better, the extent and type of injury will be unclear (sharp or blunt transection). The spectrum ranges from a lesion in continuity with potential for spontaneous recovery (focal conduction block, neurapraxia) to a transection (neurotmesis). In such cases, an observational period is indicated to monitor for spontaneous recovery. Sweating in the autonomous zone of a nerve precludes a complete lesion. If regenerative signs are insufficient after a 2- to 4-month period (adjusted to level of injury), the nerve is explored; unclear lesions in continuity are intraoperatively evaluated with nerve action potentials.[77] In conjunction with palpation and microscopic inspection, potential for spontaneous recovery is assessed. Graft reconstruction implies at least a Sunderland lesion type III with a Millesi type C fibrosis.[109,110] By means of a three-prong proximal stimulation electrode and a distal two-prong recording electrode, a test is done to see if a self-conducting compound nerve action potential can be elicited across the lesion. If a potential can be recorded, the microsurgical intervention is limited to decompression from surrounding scar and external neurolysis. If no potential can be recorded, the lesioned segment is excised and the resulting gap bridged with an interpositional nerve graft. Sometimes, only a sector of the nerve is so severely damaged that it needs graft reconstruction. If the rest of the circumference still conducts and contains healthy fascicles, a split nerve repair is indicated, which implies at least partial internal neurolysis to split the neuromatous portion from the sector with intact fascicular pattern. Graft interposition in split repairs is pleasing because the healthy nerve portion splints the graft bundle.

OUTCOMES

Outcomes depend on many different factors: the specific nerve affected, timing of repair, age of patient, level and type of lesion, and associated injuries most likely better as concomitant injuries. Reconstructive measures of nerve injury beyond 9 months have been associated with poorer results. It appears that appropriate microsurgical measures initiated in a timely manner can result in useful outcomes in more than two-thirds of cases. Seventy percent of all the iatrogenic injuries operated on in our series improved.[4] In view of the fact that that two thirds of these patients were not referred in a timely manner (delay more than 6 months post trauma), and that repairs included nerves with poorer prognosis (peroneal injury), these results should encourage attempts at early microsurgical repair. Favorable results usually can be obtained with accessory and radial nerve reconstruction. Most patients who have positioning-related nerve injuries will not require surgery. Incomplete lesions recover about 90% of the time,[85] but recovery may be lengthy. Sometimes, a good functional outcome is precluded because a patient is involved in litigation. Perioperative Parsonage-Turner syndrome is treated conservatively and has a reasonably good prognosis regarding pain and recovery of functionality. Frequently however, recovery will be incomplete and take months to years; residua like scapular winging might remain. As an adjunct to clinical examination, progress can be monitored by objective changes in MRI and electrophysiology.

MEDICOLEGAL ASPECTS

Injuries to peripheral nerves represent a sizeable proportion of medical liability cases. We assume that few of theses cases are the result of true negligence. A survey from the 1950s calculated a perioperative nerve lesion rate of 1 in 1000 operations during a 6-year period.[111] Bonney[112] remarked 22 years ago, "It is hard to know whether there has in fact been an increase in the incidence of negligence, or whether the standards by which doctors are judged have risen, or whether instances of negligence previously hidden by the enormous cost of legal action are now being revealed."

To date, the only study that specifically screened for peripheral nerve injuries among such cases evaluated the records of 2500 medical liability proceedings for the year 1984 in a former

East German county. Muller-Vahl and colleagues' analysis revealed that 638 of the cases were based on neurologic symptoms. Of these, 13% were due to direct iatrogenic damage of the involved part of the nervous system: 90% of these affected peripheral and cranial nerves and 60% of these lesions were inflicted during surgery. Injection and needle stick accounted for 22%; the remainder were due to positioning/bandage/tourniquet palsy (12%), medication (2%), radiation (1%), and other (3%). Unfortunately, longitudinal updates are not available.

It was calculated that 98.609 adverse events in 2.671863 patients occurred. Twenty-eight percent, or 27,179 of these adverse events, involved negligence.[113] Estimates based on two United States studies and one United Kingdom study suggest that negligence in the National Health Science in England may cause around 90,000 adverse events per year, involving 13,500 deaths. These adverse events apparently result in around 7000 claims (7.7% of adverse events) and 2000 payments (2.2% of adverse events).[114] The rate of nerve injuries was not extracted.

Within 4 years, from 2000 through 2003, the North German "Schlichtungsstelle" concluded 10,513 panel proceedings on medical negligence. More than 75% related to surgical and postoperative therapy. Twenty-five percent of patients claimed deficient doctor–patient communication in their initial correspondence to the panel.[115] Clearly, good communication with the patient and documentation of such conversations are important once an adverse event has occurred.

It is also obvious that precise operating room notes can be a crucial factor to support that, in fact, an injury was not the result of true negligence. Operating room notes can serve to demonstrate awareness of procedure-inherent specific risks and adequacy of preventive measures. Evident postoperative nerve damage must be addressed, treated, and likewise documented. Having records that account for presumptive diagnosis and differential, and the measures that were taken, will not only be a major step to prevent litigation, but will also inevitably lead to early and adequate therapy. Consultation with an experienced nerve surgeon is highly advisable, especially if the primary surgeon does not have enough experience with evaluation and treatment of traumatic nerve injuries.

SUMMARY

Iatrogenic nerve lesions are not infrequent; their treatment, however, is frequently inappropriate. Delayed diagnosis and referral prevail. In contrast, timely intervention has a good chance of improving the outcome. Patients benefit from early diagnosis and treatment management by a specialist in peripheral nerve surgery. Fear of litigation should not prevent proper treatment. Apart from initiation of appropriate treatment, proper documentation and communication with the patient are paramount to circumvent and confront allegations of negligence.

REFERENCES

1. Birch R, Bonney G, Parry CW. Iatropathic injury. Surgical disorders of the peripheral nerves. Edinburgh (UK): Churchill Livingstone; 1998. p. 293–333.
2. Bonney GLW. Iatropathic lesions of peripheral nerves. Curr Orthop 1997;11:255–66.
3. Khan R, Birch R. Iatropathic injuries of peripheral nerves. J Bone Joint Surg Br 2001;83(8):1145–8.
4. Kretschmer T, Antoniadis G, Braun V, et al. Evaluation of iatrogenic lesions in 722 surgically treated cases of peripheral nerve trauma. J Neurosurg 2001;94(6):905–12.
5. Kim DH, Murovic JA, Tiel R, et al. Management and outcomes in 353 surgically treated sciatic nerve lesions. J Neurosurg 2004;101(1):8–17.
6. Kim DH, Kline DG. Surgical outcome for intra- and extrapelvic femoral nerve lesions. J Neurosurg 1995;83(5):783–90.
7. Kim DH, Cho YJ, Tiel RL, et al. Surgical outcomes of 111 spinal accessory nerve injuries. Neurosurgery 2003;53(5):1106–12 [discussion: 1102–3].
8. Wilbourn AJ. Iatrogenic nerve injuries. Neurol Clin 1998;16(1):55–82.
9. Stöhr M. Iatrogene nervenläsionen. Injektion, operation, lagerung, strahlentherapie. 2nd edition. Stuttgart (Germany): Thieme; 1996.
10. Komurcu F, Zwolak P, Benditte-Klepetko H, et al. Management strategies for peripheral iatrogenic nerve lesions. Ann Plast Surg 2005;54(2):135–9 [discussion: 140–2].
11. Dellon AL. Invited discussion: management strategies for iatrogenic peripheral nerve lesions. Ann Plast Surg 2005;54(2):140–2.
12. Kretschmer T, Antoniadis G, Borm W, et al. [Iatrogenic nerve injuries. Part 1: frequency distribution, new aspects, and timing of microsurgical treatment]. Chirurg 2004;75(11):1104–12.
13. McGeorge D, Sturzenegger M, Buchler U. Tibial nerve mistakenly used as a tendon graft. Reports of three cases. J Bone Joint Surg Br 1992;74(3):365–6.
14. Geldmacher J. Median nerve as free tendon graft. Hand 1972;4(1):56.
15. Weber RV, Mackinnon SE. Median nerve mistaken for palmaris longus tendon: restoration of function with sensory nerve transfers. Hand 2007;2:1–4.

16. Oppikofer C, Tschopp H. Tibial nerve used as a tendon graft. Helv Chir Acta 1990;57:923–9.

17. Swan H, Virtue RW, Blount SG Jr, et al. Hypothermia in surgery; analysis of 100 clinical cases. Ann Surg 1955;142(3):382–400.

18. Birch R, Bonney G, Dowell J, et al. Iatrogenic injuries of peripheral nerves. J Bone Joint Surg Br 1991;73(2):280–2.

19. Tackmann W, Richter H-P, Stöhr M. Kompressionssyndrome peripherer nerven. Berlin: Springer; 1989.

20. Kretschmer T, Antoniadis G, Borm W, et al. [Pitfalls of endoscopic carpal tunnel release]. Chirurg 2004;75(12):1207–9 [in German].

21. Ferrari GP, Gilbert A. The superficial anastomosis on the palm of the hand between the ulnar and median nerves. J Hand Surg [Br] 1991;16(5):511–4.

22. Lanz U. Anatomical variations of the median nerve in the carpal tunnel. J Hand Surg [Am] 1977;2(1):44–53.

23. Stancic MF, Micovic V, Potocnjak M. The anatomy of the Berrettini branch: implications for carpal tunnel release. J Neurosurg 1999;91(6):1027–30.

24. Cannieu J. Note sur une anstomose entre la branch profonde du cubital et lemedian. Bull Soc d'Anat Physiol Bordeaux 1897;18:339–49.

25. Riche P. Le nerf cubital et les muscles de l'"eminence thenar. Bulletins et Mémoires de la Société d'Anatomie de Paris 1897;5:251–2.

26. Gruber W. Ueber die Verbindung des Nervus intermedius mit dem Nervus unaris am Unterarme des Menschen und der Saeugetiere. Archiv für Anatomie und physiologische wissenschaftliche Medizin leipzig 1870;37:501–22.

27. Lee KS, Oh CS, Chung IH, et al. An anatomic study of the Martin-Gruber anastomosis: electrodiagnostic implications. Muscle Nerve 2005;31(1):95–7.

28. Taams KO. Martin-Gruber connections in South Africa. An anatomical study. J Hand Surg [Br] 1997;22(3):328–30.

29. Martin R. Tal om Nervers allmanna Egenskaper i Manniskans Kropp. Stockholm (Sweden): L Salvius; 1763.

30. Meenakshi-Sundaram S, Sundar B, Arunkumar MJ. Marinacci communication: an electrophysiological study. Clin Neurophysiol 2003;114(12):2334–7.

31. Stancic MF, Burgic N, Micovic V. Marinacci communication. Case report. J Neurosurg 2000;92(5):860–2.

32. Marinacci A. Diagnosis of "all median hand." Bull Los Angel Neuro Soc 1964;29:191–7.

33. Kimura I, Ayyar DR, Lippmann SM. Electrophysiological verification of the ulnar to median nerve communications in the hand and forearm. Tohoku J Exp Med 1983;141(3):269–74.

34. Gutmann L. AAEM minimonograph #2: important anomalous innervations of the extremities. Muscle Nerve 1993;16(4):339–47.

35. Bazner UM, Braun V, Richter HP, et al. [Management of iatrogenic lesions of the spinal accessory nerve]. Nervenarzt 2005;76(4):462–6 [in German].

36. Bostrom D, Dahlin LB. Iatrogenic injury to the accessory nerve. Scand J Plast Reconstr Surg Hand Surg 2007;41(2):82–7.

37. Kierner AC, Zelenka I, Heller S, et al. Surgical anatomy of the spinal accessory nerve and the trapezius branches of the cervical plexus. Arch Surg 2000;135(12):1428–31.

38. Aramrattana A, Sittitrai P, Harnsiriwattanagit K. Surgical anatomy of the spinal accessory nerve in the posterior triangle of the neck. Asian J Surg 2005; 28(3):171–3.

39. Matz PG, Barbaro NM. Diagnosis and treatment of iatrogenic spinal accessory nerve injury. Am Surg 1996;62(8):682–5.

40. Coessens BC, Wood MB. Levator scapulae transfer and fascia lata fasciodesis for chronic spinal accessory nerve palsy. J Reconstr Microsurg 1995; 11(4):277–80.

41. Kim DH, Kam AC, Chandika P, et al. Surgical management and outcome in patients with radial nerve lesions. J Neurosurg 2001;95(4):573–83.

42. Hochwald NL, Levine R, Tornetta P 3rd. The risks of Kirschner wire placement in the distal radius: a comparison of techniques. J Hand Surg [Am] 1997;22(4):580–4.

43. Vernadakis AJ, Koch H, Mackinnon SE. Management of neuromas. Clin Plast Surg 2003;30(2):247–68, vii.

44. Stahl S, Rosenberg N. Surgical treatment of painful neuroma in medial antebrachial cutaneous nerve. Ann Plast Surg 2002;48(2):154–8 [discussion: 158–60].

45. Carrozzella J, Stern PJ, Von Kuster LC. Transection of radial digital nerve of the thumb during trigger release. J Hand Surg [Am] 1989;14(2 Pt 1):198–200.

46. Belkas JS, Shoichet MS, Midha R. Peripheral nerve regeneration through guidance tubes. Neurol Res 2004;26(2):151–60.

47. Archibald SJ, Krarup C, Shefner J, et al. A collagen-based nerve guide conduit for peripheral nerve repair: an electrophysiological study of nerve regeneration in rodents and nonhuman primates. J Comp Neurol 1991;306(4):685–96.

48. Mackinnon SE, Dellon AL. Clinical nerve reconstruction with a bioabsorbable polyglycolic acid tube. Plast Reconstr Surg 1990;85(3):419–24.

49. Lundborg G. Alternatives to autologous nerve grafts. Handchir Mikrochir Plast Chir 2004;36(1):1–7.

50. Dahlin LB, Lundborg G. Use of tubes in peripheral nerve repair. Neurosurg Clin N Am 2001;12(2):341–52.

51. Nahabedian MY, Dellon AL. Outcome of the operative management of nerve injuries in the ilioinguinal region. J Am Coll Surg 1997;184(3):265–8.
52. Muto CM, Pedana N, Scarpelli S, et al. Inguinal neurectomy for nerve entrapment after open/laparoscopic hernia repair using retroperitoneal endoscopic approach. Surg Endosc 2005;19(7):974–6.
53. Krahenbuhl L, Striffeler H, Baer HU, et al. Retroperitoneal endoscopic neurectomy for nerve entrapment after hernia repair. Br J Surg 1997;84(2):216–9.
54. Kim DH, Murovic JA, Tiel RL, et al. Surgical management of 33 ilioinguinal and iliohypogastric neuralgias at Louisiana State University Health Sciences Center. Neurosurgery 2005;56(5):1013–20 [discussion: 1013–20].
55. Liszka TG, Dellon AL, Manson PN. Iliohypogastric nerve entrapment following abdominoplasty. Plast Reconstr Surg 1994;93(1):181–4.
56. Ducic I, Dellon AL. Testicular pain after inguinal hernia repair: an approach to resection of the genital branch of genitofemoral nerve. J Am Coll Surg 2004;198(2):181–4.
57. Choi PD, Nath R, Mackinnon SE. Iatrogenic injury to the ilioinguinal and iliohypogastric nerves in the groin: a case report, diagnosis, and management. Ann Plast Surg 1996;37(1):60–5.
58. Schmalzried TP, Amstutz HC, Dorey FJ. Nerve palsy associated with total hip replacement. Risk factors and prognosis. J Bone Joint Surg Am 1991;73(7):1074–80.
59. Henrich M. [Sciatic nerve: special topography and possibility of injuries in surgery of the hip joint (author's transl)]. Langenbecks Arch Chir 1978;346(4):273–81 [in German].
60. Hudson AR, Hunter GA, Waddell JP. Iatrogenic femoral nerve injuries. Can J Surg 1979;22(1):62–6.
61. Schumm F, Stohr M, Bauer HL, et al. [Peripheral nerve injury due to total replacement of the hip-joint (author's transl)]. Z Orthop Ihre Grenzgeb 1975;113(6):1065–9 [in German].
62. Kahraman S, Sirin S, Erdogan E, et al. Is dysphonia permanent or temporary after anterior cervical approach? Eur Spine J 2007;16(12):2092–5.
63. Jung A, Schramm J, Lehnerdt K, et al. Recurrent laryngeal nerve palsy during anterior cervical spine surgery: a prospective study. J Neurosurg Spine 2005;2(2):123–7.
64. Brann CR, Brickley MR, Shepherd JP. Factors influencing nerve damage during lower third molar surgery. Br Dent J 1999;186(10):514–6.
65. Handschel J, Figgener L, Joos U. [Forensic evaluation of injuries to nerves and jaw bone after wisdom tooth extraction from the viewpoint of current jurisprudence]. Mund Kiefer Gesichtschir 2001;5(1):44–8 [in German].
66. Cornelius CP, Roser M, Ehrenfeld M. [Microneural reconstruction after iatrogenic lesions of the lingual nerve and the inferior alveolar nerve. Critical evaluation]. Mund Kiefer Gesichtschir 1997;1(4):213–23 [in German].
67. Kehoe NJ, Reid RP, Semple JC. Solitary benign peripheral-nerve tumours. Review of 32 years' experience. J Bone Joint Surg Br 1995;77(3):497–500.
68. Kretschmer T, Antoniadis G, Heinen C, et al. Nerve sheath tumor surgery: case-guided discussion of ambiguous findings, appropriateness of removal, repeated surgery, and nerve repairs. Neurosurg Focus 2007;22(6):E19.
69. Pandian JD, Bose S, Daniel V, et al. Nerve injuries following intramuscular injections: a clinical and neurophysiological study from Northwest India. J Peripher Nerv Syst 2006;11(2):165–71.
70. Kline DG, Kim D, Midha R, et al. Management and results of sciatic nerve injuries: a 24-year experience. J Neurosurg 1998;89(1):13–23.
71. Villarejo FJ, Pascual AM. Injection injury of the sciatic nerve (370 cases). Childs Nerv Syst 1993;9(4):229–32.
72. Fatunde OJ, Familusi JB. Injection-induced sciatic nerve injury in Nigerian children. Cent Afr J Med 2001;47(2):35–8.
73. Ohaegbulam SC. Peripheral nerve injuries from intramuscular injection of drugs. West Afr J Pharmacol Drug Res 1976;3(2):161–7.
74. Gentili F, Hudson A, Kline DG, et al. Peripheral nerve injection injury: an experimental study. Neurosurgery 1979;4(3):244–53.
75. Gentili F, Hudson AR, Kline D, et al. Early changes following injection injury of peripheral nerves. Can J Surg 1980;23(2):177–82.
76. Midha R, Guha A, Gentili F. Peripheral nerve injection injury. In: Omer G, Spinner M, Beek AV, editors. Management of peripheral nerve problems. 2nd edition. Philadelphia: WB Saunders; 1999. p. 406–13.
77. Kline D, Hudson A, Spinner R, et al. Kline & Hudson's nerve injuries. Operative results for major nerve injuries, entrapments, and tumors. 2nd edition. Philadelphia: Saunders-Elsevier; 2007.
78. Chan TY. Prolongation of prothrombin time with the use of indomethacin and warfarin. Br J Clin Pract 1997;51(3):177–8.
79. Cosma Rochat M, Waeber G, Lamy O, et al. [Oral anticoagulation and the risk of major bleeding]. Rev Med Suisse 2007;3(131):2461–2.
80. Landi A, Saracino A, Pinelli M, et al. Tourniquet paralysis in microsurgery. Ann Acad Med Singapore 1995;24(Suppl 4):89–93.
81. Levy O, David Y, Heim M, et al. Minimal tourniquet pressure to maintain arterial closure in upper limb surgery. J Hand Surg [Br] 1993;18(2):204–6.

82. Klenerman L, Biswas M, Hulands GH, et al. Systemic and local effects of the application of a tourniquet. J Bone Joint Surg Br 1980;62(3):385–8.

83. Klenerman L. Tourniquet paralysis. J Bone Joint Surg Br 1983;65(4):374–5.

84. Trojaborg W. Prolonged conduction block with axonal degeneration. An electrophysiological study. J Neurol Neurosurg Psychiatry 1977;40(1):50–7.

85. Winfree CJ, Kline DG. Intraoperative positioning nerve injuries. Surg Neurol 2005;63(1):5–18 [discussion: 18].

86. Alvine FG, Schurrer ME. Postoperative ulnar-nerve palsy. Are there predisposing factors? J Bone Joint Surg Am 1987;69(2):255–9.

87. Sawyer RJ, Richmond MN, Hickey JD, et al. Peripheral nerve injuries associated with anaesthesia. Anaesthesia 2000;55(10):980–91.

88. ASA. Practice advisory for the prevention of perioperative peripheral neuropathies: a report by the American Society of Anesthesiologists Task Force on Prevention of Perioperative Peripheral Neuropathies. Anesthesiology 2000;92(4):1168–82.

89. Rietman JS, Dijkstra PU, Hoekstra HJ, et al. Late morbidity after treatment of breast cancer in relation to daily activities and quality of life: a systematic review. Eur J Surg Oncol 2003;29(3):229–38.

90. Roth G, Magistris MR, Le Fort D, et al. [Post-radiation brachial plexopathy. Persistent conduction block. Myokymic discharges and cramps]. Rev Neurol (Paris) 1988;144(3):173–80 [in French].

91. Spillane J. Localized neuritis of the shoulder girdle: a report of 46 cases in the MEF. Lancet 1943;ii: 532–5.

92. Turner J. Neuralgic amyotrophy (paralytic brachial neuritis): with special reference to prognosis. Lancet 1957;ii:209–12.

93. Parsonage M, Turner J. Neuralgic amyotrophy: the shoulder girdle syndrome. Lancet 1948;i:973–8.

94. Malamut RI, Marques W, England JD, et al. Postsurgical idiopathic brachial neuritis. Muscle Nerve 1994;17(3):320–4.

95. Roganovic Z, Pavlicevic G. Difference in recovery potential of peripheral nerves after graft repairs. Neurosurgery 2006;59(3):621–33 [discussion: 621–33].

96. Kline DG. Surgical repair of peripheral nerve injury. Muscle Nerve 1990;13(9):843–52.

97. McAllister RM, Gilbert SE, Calder JS, et al. The epidemiology and management of upper limb peripheral nerve injuries in modern practice. J Hand Surg [Br] 1996;21(1):4–13.

98. Kline DG, Hackett ER. Reappraisal of timing for exploration of civilian peripheral nerve injuries. Surgery 1975;78(1):54–65.

99. Kandenwein JA, Kretschmer T, Engelhardt M, et al. Surgical interventions for traumatic lesions of the brachial plexus: a retrospective study of 134 cases. J Neurosurg 2005;103(4):614–21.

100. Millesi H. Reappraisal of nerve repair. Surg Clin North Am 1981;61(2):321–40.

101. Rosen B, Lundborg G. Sensory re-education after nerve repair: aspects of timing. Handchir Mikrochir Plast Chir 2004;36(1):8–12.

102. Susarla SM, Kaban LB, Donoff RB, et al. Does early repair of lingual nerve injuries improve functional sensory recovery? J Oral Maxillofac Surg 2007; 65(6):1070–6.

103. Xu QG, Zochodne DW. Ischemia and failed regeneration in chronic experimental neuromas. Brain Res 2002;946(1):24–30.

104. Ma J, Novikov LN, Kellerth JO, et al. Early nerve repair after injury to the postganglionic plexus: an experimental study of sensory and motor neuronal survival in adult rats. Scand J Plast Reconstr Surg Hand Surg 2003;37(1):1–9.

105. McKay Hart A, Brannstrom T, Wiberg M, et al. Primary sensory neurons and satellite cells after peripheral axotomy in the adult rat: timecourse of cell death and elimination. Exp Brain Res 2002; 142(3):308–18.

106. West CA, Davies KA, Hart AM, et al. Volumetric magnetic resonance imaging of dorsal root ganglia for the objective quantitative assessment of neuron death after peripheral nerve injury. Exp Neurol 2007;203(1):22–33.

107. Terenghi G, Calder JS, Birch R, et al. A morphological study of Schwann cells and axonal regeneration in chronically transected human peripheral nerves. J Hand Surg [Br] 1998;23(5):583–7.

108. Ma J, Novikov LN, Wiberg M, et al. Delayed loss of spinal motoneurons after peripheral nerve injury in adult rats: a quantitative morphological study. Exp Brain Res 2001;139(2):216–23.

109. Sunderland S. Nerves and nerve injuries. 2nd edition. Edinburgh (UK): Churchill Livingstone; 1978.

110. Millesi H, Rath T, Reihsner R, et al. Microsurgical neurolysis: it's anatomical and physiological basis and classification. Microsurgery 1993;14:430–9.

111. Dhuner K. Nerve injuries following operations: surveys of cases occurring during a 6 year period. Anesthesiology 1950;11:289–93.

112. Bonney G. Iatrogenic injuries of nerves. J Bone Joint Surg Br 1986;68(1):9–13.

113. Brennan TA, Leape LL, Laird NM, et al. Incidence of adverse events and negligence in hospitalized patients. Results of the Harvard Medical Practice Study I. N Engl J Med 1991;324(6):370–6.

114. Towse A, Danzon P. Medical negligence and the NHS: an economic analysis. Health Econ 1999; 8(2):93–101.

115. Neu J, Scheppokat KD, Vinz H. [Medical risk and iatrogenic injury–"accident reports" from the North German Schlichtungsstelle (expert panel for extrajudicial claims resolution)]. Z Arztl Fortbild Qualitatssich 2004;98(7):567–74.

Nerve Tubes for Peripheral Nerve Repair

Godard C.W. de Ruiter, MD[a], Robert J. Spinner, MD[b,c],
Michael J. Yaszemski, MD, PhD[c], Anthony J. Windebank, MD[d],
Martijn J.A. Malessy, MD, PhD[a],*

KEYWORDS

- Nerve tubes • Nerve guides • Nerve conduits
- Animal models • Evaluation methods
- Clinical nerve repair • Modified nerve tubes

At this moment, the gold standard for repair of nerve defects that cannot be directly restored without tension to the nerve ends is still the autologous nerve graft (**Fig. 1**A). Most commonly, the sural nerve is used, taken from the leg of the patient. Obviously, repair with autografts has several disadvantages, such as the need for an extra incision, limited availability, mismatch in size of the damaged nerve and the donor nerve, and the chance for the development of a painful neuroma. Because of these disadvantages, various alternatives have been developed for autograft repair (eg, repair with autogenous venous grafts[1] and nerve allografts,[2,3] and nerve tubes, guides, or conduits). Practical advantages of nerve tubes are the unlimited right-off-the-shelf availability in different sizes that match the damaged nerve (**Fig. 1**B). Besides, functional recovery is often reduced after autograft repair compared with direct coaptation repair. A possible explanation is that axons need to cross two coaptation sites, which might decrease the number of axons reaching the distal targets and lead to increased misdirection of regenerating axons.[4] An ideal alternative, therefore, will also lead to improved regeneration and functional results of nerve repair. In this article, the authors give an overview of the current experimental and clinical data on nerve tubes for peripheral nerve repair. The goal of this article is not to be complete but to provide an overview of the nerve tube literature and to analyze critically the data on which the step from laboratory to clinical use is based.

DEVELOPMENT OF NERVE TUBES
The Concept of Nerve Tube Repair

The first attempts at nerve tube, entubulation, or tubulization repair date back to the end of the nineteenth century (see Table 1 in the article by Weiss elsewhere in this issue).[5] The results of these first attempts were disappointing and later viewed by Sunderland[6] as only of historical interest. The concept of the nerve tube was reintroduced in the 1980s, mainly as a tool to investigate the process of regeneration. In the beginning, silicone tubes were used mostly. Later, nerve tubes of other synthetic nonbiodegradable[7–11] and biodegradable materials (including polymers of glycolic and lactic acid,[12–14] and caprolactone[15,16]) were developed. These first experiments with silicone nerve tubes by Lundborg and colleagues[17] demonstrated that axons can successfully regenerate across a 1-cm gap in the rat sciatic nerve model. No regeneration was observed in the absence of the distal nerve stump and across 15-mm defects, which was later explained by the accumulation of neurotrophic factors in the silicone chamber that

[a] Department of Neurosurgery, Leiden University Medical Center, Leiden, The Netherlands
[b] Department of Neurologic Surgery, Mayo Clinic, Rochester, MN, USA
[c] Department of Orthopedic Surgery, Mayo Clinic, Rochester, MN, USA
[d] Department of Neurology, Mayo Clinic, Rochester, MN, USA
* Corresponding author.
E-mail address: M.J.A.Malessy@lumc.nl (M.J.A. Malessy).

Neurosurg Clin N Am 20 (2009) 91–105
doi:10.1016/j.nec.2008.08.001
1042-3680/08/$ – see front matter © 2008 Elsevier Inc. All rights reserved.

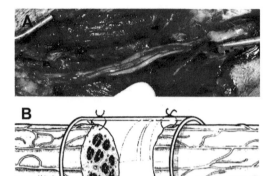

Fig. 1. (A) Repair of a radial nerve lesion (after a humerus fracture) with autologous sural nerve grafts. (B) Nerve tube repair. (*Adapted from* Lundborg G, Dahlin LB, Danielsen N. Ulnar nerve repair by the silicone chamber technique: case report. Scand J Plast Reconstr Hand Surg 1991;25:79–82; with permission.)

probably only act over a limited distance (neurotropism or chemotaxis). Another explanation might be that the formation of a fibrin matrix (**Fig. 2**), which is essential in the process of regeneration,[18] does not occur if the gap is too long.[19]

Physical Characteristics of the Nerve Tube

Other physical properties, including the dimensions of the nerve tube, prefilling with phosphate-buffered saline (PBS),[20] and porosity,[19] have also been shown to affect the formation of the fibrin matrix. Jenq and Coggeshall[21,22] found that the addition of holes to silicone nerve tubes increased the number of myelinated axons and the length of the gap that could be bridged. Possible explanations were that by adding holes, cells (eg, macrophages and leucocytes) and molecules (eg, fibrin and fibronectin) involved in the formation of the fibrin matrix could enter the site of regeneration. The importance of the permeability of the nerve tube was later confirmed in other experiments,[15,23–26] although what the ideal pore size is exactly (microporous or macroporous) still remains questionable. Disadvantages of macropores might be that neurotrophic factors can diffuse out of the nerve tube and that the fibrin matrix might be disorganized (orientation perpendicular to the pores instead of longitudinal). Permeability not only depends on pore size but may also be affected by, for example, hydrophilic properties of the material. Next to permeability, the surface texture and dimensions of the nerve tube have been found to affect the formation of the fibrin matrix;[8] with smooth surfaces (eg, in silicone nerve tubes), the

longitudinal matrix coalesces and forms a free-floating nerve cable, whereas with rough surfaces, the tissue disperses and completely fills the lumen of the nerve tube.[27]

With the potential use of nerve tubes, especially biodegradable nerve tubes, for clinical nerve repair, other physical characteristics were also investigated, including swelling and degradation properties. Swelling of a nerve tube might primarily block the lumen for regeneration or might secondarily lead to compression of the regenerated nerve. Degradation may cause swelling owing to the accumulation of degradation products that can increase the osmotic pressure in the tube.[16,28] Besides, degradation products might be toxic or might interfere with the process of regeneration. Degradation may also, in time, affect the porosity and tensile properties of the nerve tube. These tensile properties are important because a nerve tube should be flexible for implantation into mobile limbs but at the same time, the nerve tube should be resistant to deformation (elongation, breaking, or kinking) and strong enough to hold a suture. Transparency is preferred for suturing and accurate positioning of the nerve stumps. In the end, nerve tubes must be sterilizable without compromising the physical properties mentioned above. **Table 1** summarizes the known physical properties of some of the frequently used nerve tubes. It is important to note the physical properties of the nerve tube depend not only on the biomaterial but also on other factors, such as the dimensions of the nerve tube and fabrication technique. Not all nerve tubes that are currently available for clinical use have been characterized extensively in vitro before clinical application.

Evaluation Methods and Animal Models

Different evaluation methods and animal models have been used to investigate the process of regeneration across nerve tubes. Most experiments have been performed in the rat sciatic nerve model. Commonly used evaluation methods in this model include electrophysiology, nerve morphometry, and walking track analysis (see **Table 1**). The first, most important observation, however, is the percentage of successful regeneration across the nerve tube. Failures due to collapse, swelling, and suture pullout have been reported.[12,14,29,30] The second most important observation is the quantity of regeneration across the nerve tube. This quantity is mostly determined for the number of axons (myelinated or unmyelinated) at the middle part or distal to the nerve tube and is then preferably compared with the numbers in normal nerve and after autograft repair. However, the numbers

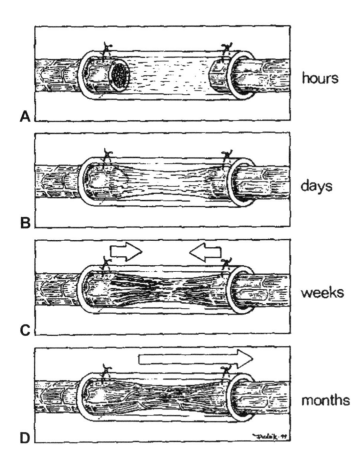

hours

A

days

B

weeks

C

months

D

Fig. 2. The different phases in the process of regeneration across the nerve tube. (*A*) Within hours of implantation, the lumen fills with fluid containing neurotrophic factors and various inflammatory cells. (*B*) Within days, a fibrin matrix is formed between the nerve stumps. (*C*) In weeks, Schwann cells, fibroblasts, and microvessels migrate along the fibrin matrix from both proximal and distal nerve ends. (*D*) In months, axons regenerate from the proximal nerve stump into the matrix. (*From* Dahlin L, Lundborg G. Use of tubes in peripheral nerve repair. Neurosurg Clin N Am 2000;12(2):341–52; with permission.)

of axons that have been reported in the literature differ.[31] Sometimes only the density of nerve fibers in a specified area is provided (see **Table 1**).[32,33] This area may not be representative of the total cross-sectional area of the nerve. Also, the total number of axons may not be the best parameter to quantify regeneration, because this number is increased early in the process of regeneration because of collateral sprouting or branching, and has been found to decrease later.[34] Different factors may stimulate the sprouting or branching of axons (eg, the addition of Schwann cells[35–37] or neurotrophic factors). Numbers may increase without an actual increase in the number of motoneurons and dorsal root ganglion cells from which axons have regenerated across the nerve tube. In the authors' opinion, quantification of regeneration across the nerve tube can therefore best be performed with retrograde tracing. The technique with fluorescent dyes that are retrogradely transported to the motoneuron or dorsal root ganglion can also be used to analyze the accuracy of regeneration across the nerve tube. For example, different tracers can be applied sequentially to the same nerve branch before and after nerve repair to determine the direction of regenerating axons, or simultaneously to different nerve branches (eg, the tibial and peroneal nerves) to determine the dispersion of regenerating axons across the nerve tube.[38] Although it has often been suggested that nerve tube repair leads to an improved orientation of regenerating nerve fibers, only a few studies have actually investigated the accuracy of regeneration across the nerve tube.[39–43] These studies did not show an improved accuracy after nerve tube repair compared with direct coaptation or autograft repair. Brushart and colleagues[44] actually found that regenerating axons might disperse across the tube and that this dispersion increases with gap length. This dispersion of regenerating axons might lead to (1) misdirection of regenerating axons or (2) polyinnervation of different targets by axons originating from the same neuron. In comparison, autograft

Table 1
Experimental data on some of the frequently used nerve tubes

	Nerve Tube				Model			Evaluation		
Material	Permeability	Flexibility[a]	Degradation	Swelling	Animal	Nerve	Gap Size	Methods	Control	Follow-Up
Natural										
Collagen[53,54,116]	Diffusion of molecules up to 215 Å	—	—	3 × dry weight	Monkeys Rats	Median Sciatic	4, 5 mm 4 mm	Number of axons, electrophysiology Electrophysiology	Reversed autograft and normal, direct coaptation, and negative controls	Up to 760 d 4 and 12 wk
Synthetic										
Nonbiodegradable										
Silicone[17]	—	—	—	—	Rat	Sciatic	6, 10, 15, 20 mm	Nerve histology	Absence distal nerve stump	1 mo
Hydrogel, p(HEMA-co-MMA) 86:14[b,29,117]	c	—	—	—	Rat	Sciatic	10 mm	Percentages successful regeneration, nerve morphometry	Isografts	8 and 16 wk
Biodegradable										
PGA[33]	—	—	—	—	Monkeys	Ulnar	3 cm	Electrophysiology, nerve fiber density	Sural nerve grafts	1 y
PLA[118]	83.5%, 12.1 μm[d]	80 MPa 1.0 MPa	Mn 43% at 8 wk	—	Rats	Sciatic	1 cm	SFI, gastrocnemius muscle weight, nerve fiber density	Reversed isograft	16 wk
PLGA,[119] 75:25	83%, 20 μm[d]	8 MPa 0.95 MPa	Mn 38% at 8 wk	—	—	—	—	—	—	—

PLC,[15,120] 50:50	Low and high[e]	3 MPa 25 MPa	Mn 50% at 10 mo	—	Mice	Sciatic	6 mm	Percentages successful reinnervation, number of axons, electrophysiology, sweating tests	Silicone, Teflon, collagen, polysulfone	4, 5 mo
					Rats	Sciatic	8 mm	Simultaneous retrograde tracing, electrophysiology, SFI	Normal, autograft, silicone	90 d
PLC,[32,121,122] 50:50 (DL 85:15)	2.5 MPa[f]	45% mass loss at 8 mo	300% volume increase at 3 mo	Rats	Sciatic	1 cm[32] 15 mm[122]	Nerve fiber density Electrophysiology, video analysis	Reversed autograft	10 wk 5 mo
TMC-CL,[123] 50:50	No pores[g]	23.5 MPa 1 MPa	—	—	—	—	—	—	—

Abbreviations: DL, L (left) and D (Dexter) lactides; HEMA-co-MMA, hydroxyethyl methacrylate-co-methyl methacrylate Mn, average molecular weight; MPa, megapascal; PGA, poly-glycolic acid; PLA, poly(L-lactic acid); PLC, poly(DL-lactide-ε-caprolactone); PLGA, poly (DL-lactic co-glycolic acid); SFI, sciatic function index; TMC-CL, trimethylene carbonate-co-ε-caprolactone.

a Elastic modulus, tensile strength.
b Poly(2-hydroxyethyl methacrylate-co-methyl methacrylate).
c Depending on ratio HEMA:MMA, microporous and macroporous determined with surface electron microscopy.[119]
d Porosity and mean pore size, measured by mercury porosimetry.[119]
e Low prepared with fine powder of amylose (<10 μm), high with glucose of around 10 μm; permeability tested with ultraviolet spectroscopy.[121]
f Rapid loss after 3 weeks.[121]
g But slow diffusion of methylene blue molecules, analyzed with ultraviolet spectroscopy.

repair contains more regenerating branched axons to the inside of the basal lamina tubes.[45]

Functional analysis is ultimately the most important method for translating the results of nerve tube repair into patients. This type of analysis has not often been included in the evaluation of nerve tube repair. The reason might be that the most commonly used method, the sciatic function index (SFI), is based on footprint analysis[46,47] and lacks sensitivity, which might be because of contractures[48] and autotomy[49] but also because the SFI evaluates the distal foot muscles that often do not recover because of the prolonged time of denervation.[50] The authors, therefore, recently introduced the use of two-dimensional motion analysis to measure the recovery of more proximally located muscles from the ankle angles of maximum plantar and dorsiflexion during the stance and swing phases.[51] This method was found to be more sensitive than the SFI and is currently being used by their laboratory for functional analysis after different nerve repair techniques. Another advantage of functional analysis in comparison with other evaluation methods is that animals can be evaluated at multiple time points. Combined with electrophysiology, this method can provide insight into the time to reinnervation and recovery.

Electrophysiology is frequently included in the evaluation of results after nerve tube repair. Most often, compound muscle action potentials (CMAPs) are recorded and analyzed for amplitude, area under the curve, or latency.[31] This method is not as time consuming as most other evaluation methods, but it should not be used instead of functional evaluation. CMAP recovery after nerve repair may be better than functional recovery because of distal sprouting, which results in larger motor units, and because of misdirected axons that contribute to the CMAP but probably not to recovery of function.[54]

Different animal models have also been used for the analysis of nerve tube repair, including mice, rabbits, and monkeys (see **Table 1**). The disadvantage of this use of larger animal models is that it makes it difficult to compare the results between studies, especially the extrapolation of the size of the nerve gap.[52] An obvious advantage of larger animals is the closer-to-human comparison, especially for the primate model. The polyglycolic acid (PGA) and collagen nerve tube (which are now available for clinical use, see later discussion) were first investigated experimentally in monkeys.[33,53,54] In 1988, Dellon and Mackinnon[33] published the first study in which they compared repair of a 3-cm gap in the ulnar nerve (proximal to the elbow) in adult male *Macaca cynomolgus* monkeys

with sural nerve grafts and solid and mesh PGA tubes (eight repairs per group). After 1 year of follow-up, nerve fiber densities did not differ from normal after the different repair techniques. Unfortunately, absolute numbers of nerve fibers were not provided. Electromyography demonstrated recovery in 19 out of 28 (68%) of the intrinsic muscles studied in the solid and mesh tube groups (2 muscles per repair, seven repairs per group). Recovery after autograft repair was not reported because the Martin-Gruber anastomosis in this group had not been divided. Electromyography results were reported for 7 tube repairs, because one case of solid tube repair had no continuity (the reason for exclusion of one of the mesh tubes was not reported). In three out of seven solid and four out of eight mesh tubes, some scar tissue was observed in the center of the tube. Later, the same investigators published another study performed in monkeys, in which regeneration across 2- and 5-cm nerve gaps in radial sensory and ulnar nerves was compared for crimped and mesh glycolide trimethylene carbonate (Maxon) and collagen nerve tubes.[55] Poor regeneration was found in that study[55] across 5-cm nerve gaps.

Archibald and colleagues[53] compared repair of 4-mm gaps with collagen nerve tubes and autografts (reversed segments) in rats (sciatic nerve) and *Macaca fascicularis* monkeys (median nerve, 2 cm above the wrist). This study showed that collagen nerve tube repair was as effective as autograft repair in terms of physiologic responses from target muscle and sensory nerves. Later, they reported a second study on collagen nerve tube repair of 5-mm gap median nerve lesions (again, 2 cm above the wrist) in monkeys, which included 3 years of electrophysiologic assessment and nerve morphometry.[54] In this study, a significantly increased number of axons distal to the repair site (1.2 to 2 times larger) was found after both collagen nerve tube and autograft repair.

CLINICAL USE OF NERVE TUBES FOR PERIPHERAL NERVE REPAIR

Currently, various nerve tubes are available for clinical nerve repair: Neurotube (PGA), Neuragen (collagen), Neurolac (polycaprolactone), Neuro-Matrix and Neuroflex (both collagen), and SaluBridge (hydrogel, nonbiodegradable).[56] These nerve tubes are mainly used in the repair of small nerve gaps (<3 cm) in small sensory nerves, such as digital nerve lesions. In addition, recently a processed allograft (Avance) has become available for clinical use. In this article, the authors only discuss the results of the large series and randomized studies that have been reported on the clinical use of the silicone, PGA, and poly(DL-lactide-ε-caprolactone) (PLC) nerve tubes. In addition, series have been reported on the use of nonbiodegradable polytetrafluoroethylene (PTFE) nerve tubes (GORE-TEX or Teflon) for median and ulnar nerve[57] and inferior alveolar/lingual nerve lesions,[58,59] a small series on the use of collagen (Neuragen) nerve tubes in the repair of obstetric brachial plexus injuries,[60] and several cases on the use of PGA nerve tubes (for the repair of the inferior alveolar nerve,[61] medial plantar nerve,[62] zygomatic and buccinatory branches of the facial nerve,[63] and spinal accessory nerve;[64] for nerve reconstruction after a hallux-to-thumb transfer;[65] and for interfascicular median nerve repair with multiple PGA tubes).[66] Combinations of PGA tubes with collagen sponges[67,68] and an interposed nerve segment[69] have also been used in patients, and a chitosan tube with internal oriented filaments of PGA[70] (see section on modifications to the common hollow nerve tube).

Silicone Nerve Tubes

In 1997, Lundborg and colleagues[71] published their first results of 1-year follow-up of a prospective randomized study, in which small defects (3–4 mm) after fresh and complete clean-cut transection of the ulnar and median nerves proximal to the wrist (up to 10 cm) were repaired with silicone nerve tubes (11 patients) or conventional microsurgical direct coaptation repair (8 patients). Several tests were used to evaluate the results (see **Table 2**). In general, no significant differences were found between the two types of repair. Also in the 5-year follow-up (2004),[72] no significant difference in outcome was found, except for significantly less cold intolerance after silicone nerve tube repair. The use of silicone nerve tubes, however, has been heavily criticized,[73,74] mainly because of the potential late compression of the nerve by the nonbiodegradable tube. Critics often refer to a study by Merle and colleagues,[75] in which silicone tube (1 patient) and sheath repair (2 patients) resulted in chronic nerve compression. In addition, a study by Braga-Silva[76] was reported on silicone nerve tube repair of median and ulnar nerve lesions (up to 3 cm) in which 7 out of 26 patients requested removal of the nerve tube because of local discomfort. Dahlin and Lundborg[77] themselves performed a re-exploration surgery in 7 patients, as an ethically permitted part of their prospective study (4 patients complained of local discomfort), but found no signs of neuroma and only a mild microscopic foreign body reaction in 2 cases. After removal of the silicone nerve tube, no new impairment of nerve function occurred. They emphasized that in their studies, silicone nerve tubes were used with a diameter exceeding the diameter of the nerve by at least 30%. Nevertheless, they acknowledged that a biodegradable nerve tube would be better, provided that it degrades with minimal tissue reaction and without impairment of nerve regeneration.[78]

Polyglycolic Acid Nerve Tubes

In 2000, Weber and colleagues[79] presented the results of the first multicenter randomized study on the repair of digital nerves with gaps up to 3 cm using glycolic acid (PGA) nerve tubes. Ten years before that, Mackinnon and Dellon[80] had already presented a series of 15 patients in which they had also used PGA nerve tubes to repair digital nerve defects up to 3 cm. In that study, excellent results were reported for 5 patients (33%), good results for 8 patients (53%), and poor results for 2 patients (14%). In the randomized study by Weber and colleagues,[79] PGA nerve tube repair was compared with standard repair (direct coaptation for gaps less than 8 mm and nerve graft repair for gaps greater than 8 mm). The overall results at 1-year follow-up showed no significant difference between the two groups, with excellent and good outcome in respectively 44% and 30% of the repairs with PGA nerve tubes compared with 43% of both excellent and good outcome after standard repairs. The investigators subsequently performed a subgroup analysis for different gap lengths ($\leq$4 mm, 5–7 mm, and 8 mm–3 cm) that demonstrated excellent results for gaps less than or equal to 4 mm for moving two-point discrimination (m2PD) in 91% of PGA nerve tube repairs compared with 49% of standard repairs ($P =$ .02). As noted by Lundborg in the discussion on this article, the statistics of this study are difficult to interpret because of the heterogeneous data (eg, different levels of injury and mechanisms of injury were included). Also, the numbers per group of PGA nerve tube and standard repair for subgroup analysis were not provided. However, it is not clear why separate subgroup analysis was performed for gaps less than or equal to 4 mm. Although the investigators mention that it is generally accepted that 4 mm is the maximum gap length for digital nerves to be repaired with minimal tension by the end-to-end method, in the standard repair group all gaps of 5 to 7 mm were repaired by direct coaptation. In the 5- to 7-mm gap group, excellent results were obtained in only 17% of the PGA nerve tube repairs and 57% of the standard repairs ($P =$ .06). The technique used to measure two-point discrimination was not based on the Moberg

Table 2
Clinical data on the use of nerve tubes in large series and randomized controlled clinical trials

		Nerve Tube					Evaluation			
Material	First Author (y)	Study Type	Numbers	Patient Age (y)	Nerves, Location	Gap Size	Methods	Control	Interval	Follow-Up Period
Synthetic										
Nonbiodegradable										
Silicone	Lundborg (1997)[71]	RCT	11 patients, 8 controls	12–72, mean 29	Median and ulnar, <10 cm proximal	3–4 mm	Tactilometry, s2PD, m2PD, and strength abduction dig its I and II[a]	Direct repair	No	1 y
	Lundborg (2004)[72]	RCT	17 patients, 13 controls	12–72, mean 32		3–5 mm	Model instrument for outcome after nerve repair,[124] neurophysiology			5 y
Biodegradable										
Polyglycolic acid	Mackinnon (1990)[80]	Series	15 patients, 16 repairs	30.5 (SD 7.6)	Digital	0.5–3.0 cm, mean 1.7	s2PD and m2PD: Excellent[c]: ≤6 mm and ≤3 mm Good: 7–15 mm and 4–7 mm Poor: ≥15 mm and ≥7 mm	No	None placed acutely	11–32 mo, mean 22.4
	Weber (2000)[79]	RCMT	62 repairs, 74 controls	17–65, mean 35	Digital, distal to wrist	7.0 mm,[b] control 4.3		Gap <8 mm direct repair; Gap >8 mm nerve graft	50 <72 h; 54–20 d; 7 >20 d	Mean 9.4 mo, Control 8.1
	Battiston (2005)[82]	Series	19	15–67, mean 40	Digital	1.0–4.0 cm, mean 2.0	s2PD and m2PD, MRC, quick-DASH	Muscle-vein combined conduits	Primary: 16 mo	6–74 mo, mean 30
PLC	Bertleff (2005)[83]	RCMT	21, 13 controls	Mean 43	Digital, distal to wrist	Up to 2.0 cm	s2PD and m2PD	Direct repair	Not provided	1 y

Abbreviations: m2PD, moving two-point discrimination; MRC, strength for British Medical Research Council scale; PLC, poly(DL-lactide-ε-caprolactone); quick-DASH, disabilities of the arm, shoulder, and hand; RCMT, randomized controlled multicenter trial; RCT, randomized controlled clinical trial; s2PD, static two-point discrimination; SD, standard deviation.
a Tactilometry for perception of vibration was measured with Semmes-Weinstein monofilaments, s2PD and m2PD were measured using Moberg's method,[81] and the strength of abduction digits I and II was measured with an intrinsicmeter. In addition, the presence of a neuroma, hyperesthesia, and cold intolerance were noted.
b A gap of 5 mm was left intentionally, even in defects of 0 to 4 mm.
c In Weber study, outcome was defined for the lower of the s2PD or m2PD, as defined in the study by Mackinnon and Dellon, except that excellent outcome was defined for m2PD less than or equal to 4 mm.

approach,[81] with application of light pressure (just enough to blanch the skin), but with increasing pressure until the stimulus was perceived by the patient (see discussion by Lundborg).

Another large series on PGA nerve tube repairs of 19 digital nerves in 17 patients who had gaps up to 4 cm was published in 2005 by Battiston and colleagues.[82] In this study, very good results (S3+ and S4, defined for static two-point discrimination [s2PD] up to 15 mm) were reported for 13 patients (76.5%) and good results in 3 patients (17.7%). Analysis of the data, however, shows that in only 2 patients, S4 (s2PD 2–6 mm) was obtained and that no results were excellent for m2PD (≤3 mm, by the definition used in the studies by Mackinnon[80] and Weber;[79] see **Table 2**), and good results were obtained (m2PD 4–7 mm) in only 4 out of 19 repairs.

In conclusion, PGA nerve tubes might lead to results comparable to conventional nerve repair in the repair of small gaps in digital nerve lesions, but care should be taken with the interpretation of the data and the wide application to the repair of other nerve lesions based on these results.

Poly(DL-Lactide-ε-Caprolactone) Nerve Tubes

In 2003, Bertleff and colleagues[83] presented the results of a multicenter trial on digital nerve repair for gaps up to 2 cm that compared PLC nerve tube and standard repair, which were all direct coaptation repairs (with the finger flexed to reduce tension). Randomization was performed separately for gaps less than or equal to 4 mm, 4 to 8 mm, and 8 to 20 mm. Sensory recovery was evaluated at 3, 6, 9, and 12 months for the s2PD and m2PD measured with the pressure-specified sensory device.[84] Two-point discrimination for PLC and direct coaptation repair of gaps up to 2 cm showed no significant differences, but unfortunately, results for subgroup analysis were not provided. The pressure that was applied (to feel the stimulus) seemed larger in the PLC nerve tube repair group than in the direct repair group.[83] More wound healing problems were observed after PLC nerve tube repair than after direct coaptation. In a recent review, Meek and colleagues[85] also commented that small fragments of biomaterial in experiments with PLC nerve tubes were still found 24 months after implantation and that PLC nerve tubes are normally stiff and only flexible after putting in warm saline before implantation. A more extensive report on the use of PLC nerve tubes (according to the investigators) will soon be published.[85] So far, ample evidence supports the clinical use of PLC tubes.

Conclusion: Clinical Use Nerve Tubes

In conclusion, in the authors' opinion at this moment, care should be taken with the wide use of tubes in peripheral nerve repair, not only because of the concerns mentioned above but also because of the following reasons. First, little is still known about the accuracy of regeneration across nerve tubes. In the repair of larger mixed or motor nerves, dispersion of regenerating axons across the nerve tube may lead to misdirection and polyinnervation (see section on the development of nerve tubes) and result in impaired functional recovery because of, for example, cocontraction or synkinesis. In most experimental studies on nerve tube repair, accuracy of regeneration and functional analysis were not included. Finally, not all nerve tubes that are now available for clinical use have been characterized extensively in vitro and the long-term effects of biodegradable nerve tubes have not (yet) been reported (see **Table 2**, follow-up studies 1–2 years).

MODIFICATIONS TO THE HOLLOW NERVE TUBE

Different modifications to the common hollow or single lumen nerve tube have been investigated to enhance regeneration and extend the gap that can be bridged (**Fig. 3**). Prefilling of the nerve tubes with PBS and the addition of pores have already been mentioned in the section on the development of nerve tubes. In the following section, the authors briefly discuss the addition of different extracellular molecules (collagen and laminin), internal frameworks, supportive cells, and nerve growth factors.

Collagen and Laminin-Containing Gels

Collagen and laminin are involved in the process of regeneration by forming a substrate for the migration of nonneuronal cells. Filling of silicone nerve tubes with collagen and laminin-containing gels has been shown to increase the rate of regeneration[11] and the gap that can be bridged (up to 15–20 mm).[86] This effect, however, depends on several factors, including the concentration[87] and the permeability of the nerve tube.[88] Alignment of the collagen (gravitational or magnetic) may also further enhance regeneration.[89] Currently, different collagen and laminin-containing gels (eg, BD Matrigel) are being used for the incorporation of supportive cells and growth factors.[37,90,91] Also, oligopeptides derived from laminin-integrin active sites are being investigated for a potential role in the guidance of regenerating axons.[92]

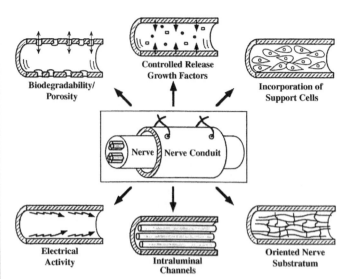

Fig. 3. Different modifications to the single lumen nerve tube or conduit. (*From* Hudson TW, Evans GR, Schmidt CE. Engineering strategies for peripheral nerve repair. Clin Plast Surg 1999;26:617–28; with permission.)

Internal Framework

An intrinsic framework may also enhance regeneration and increase the gap that can be bridged because of stabilization of the fibrin matrix that is formed inside the nerve tube. Different internal structures have been investigated, including polyamide filaments,[93] laminin-coated fibers,[94] PGA filaments,[95] and collagen sponges.[94,96] The combinations of PGA tube and collagen sponge, and chitosan tube and PGA filaments, have already been used clinically, although little information exists on the effect of these internal structures on the accuracy of regeneration. Different tissues have also been added to the nerve tube (eg, interposed nerve segments[97] and denatured muscle).[98] In addition, nerve tubes with a modified microarchitecture have been developed. Yoshii and colleagues[99] developed a scaffold of longitudinally orientated collagen filaments that has been shown to lead to successful regeneration across gaps of 20 mm and even 30 mm in rats.[100] Another example of a modification to the common single lumen nerve tube structure is the multichannel nerve tube structure.[28,38,101–104] This structure has several advantages: It provides more surface area for cell attachment and controlled release of incorporated growth factors, and may reduce dispersion by containment of axonal branches, as in the autografts consisting of multiple basal lamina tubes.[39]

Supportive Cells

The addition of Schwann cells to the nerve tube has also been found to enhance regeneration in small gaps[36,37,90] and to extend the gap that can

be bridged to about 2 cm,[35,91] although, remarkably, autograft repair in most studies still was found to be superior.[37,90,91,105,106] Schwann cells possibly stimulate regeneration by the production of a range of growth factors and extracellular molecules (laminin), and may play a mechanical role by forming a cable bridging the gap.[37] Schwann cells can also be genetically modified to overexpress certain growth factors. A disadvantage of the addition of Schwann cells is that it still requires the explantation of a donor nerve, to isolate autologous Schwann cells weeks before reconstruction. This disadvantage may be overcome in the future by the differentiation of, for example, bone marrow stem cells into Schwann cells.[107]

Growth Factors

The addition of different growth factors to the nerve tube, including nerve growth factor, glial cell derived neurotrophic factor, brain-derived neurotrophic factor, and fibroblast growth factor, has also been shown to enhance regeneration and increase the nerve gap that can be bridged (to 15 mm). These growth factors can be added directly to the tube (into a solution)[108] or can be released after absorption to fibronectin mats,[109,110] collagen matrices,[30] bovine serum albumin or from delivery systems such as subcutaneous minipumps[111] or microspheres that are incorporated during the fabrication process of the nerve tube.[112,113] The advantage of growth factors in comparison to Schwann cells is that no extra procedure is needed. The advantage of delivery of growth factors from microspheres is the potential for controlled release over an extended period of time without leakage from the tube.

Conductive Polymers

Finally, conductive polymers may also enhance regeneration across the nerve tube. Aebischer and colleagues[114] found significantly increased numbers of myelinated axons after repair with poled versus unpoled polyvinylidene fluoride tubes, possibly by accelerated axonal elongation on the charged surface. Schmidt and colleagues[115] found an almost twofold neurite outgrowth in vitro on conductive polypyrrole films after electric stimulation.

SUMMARY

In this article, the authors provided an overview of the experimental and clinical data currently available on the use of nerve tubes for peripheral nerve repair. At present, no sound scientific proof exists of the superiority of the empty hollow biodegradable nerve tubes that are now clinically used, as compared with direct coaptation or autograft repair. The repair of all sorts of nerve lesions may lead to unnecessary failures and, again, a discontinuation of interest in the concept of the nerve tube. The extensions of the applications, especially in the repair of larger mixed or motor nerves, should be carefully evaluated. Also, although the autologous nerve graft has several practical disadvantages, it still has several advantages, such as the presence of Schwann cells that secrete growth factors and basal lamina tubes that contain regenerating axons, besides the favorable properties of the natural strength and flexibility of the nerve, and the fact that it is immunocompatible. Eventually, different modifications to the single lumen nerve tube might lead to a nerve tube that is a better alternative than autologous nerve graft repair.

ACKNOWLEDGMENT

The authors appreciate the assistance of Dr. Huan Wang.

REFERENCES

1. Chiu DT, Janecka I, Krizek TJ, et al. Autogenous vein graft as a conduit for nerve regeneration. Surgery 1982;91(2):226–33.
2. Mackinnon SE, Doolabh VB, Novak CB, et al. Clinical outcome following nerve allograft transplantation. Plast Reconstr Surg 2001;107(6):1419–29.
3. Siemionow M, Sonmez E. Nerve allograft transplantation: a review. J Reconstr Microsurg 2007;23(8):511–20.
4. de Ruiter GC, Malessy MJ, Alaid AO, et al. Misdirection of regenerating motor axons after nerve injury and repair in the rat sciatic nerve model. Exp Neurol 2008;211(2):339–50.
5. Weiss P. The technology of nerve regeneration: a review. Sutureless tubulation and related methods for nerve repair. J Neurosurg 1944;1:400–50.
6. Sunderland S. Nerve grafting. Edinburgh, London, New York: Churchill, Livingstone; 1978.
7. Uzman BG, Villegas GM. Mouse sciatic nerve regeneration through semipermeable tubes: a quantitative model. J Neurosci Res 1983;9(3):325–38.
8. Aebischer P, Guenard V, Valentini RF. The morphology of regenerating peripheral nerves is modulated by the surface microgeometry of polymeric guidance channels. Brain Res 1990;531(1–2):211–8.
9. Scaravilli F. Regeneration of the perineurium across a surgically induced gap in a nerve encased in a plastic tube. J Anat 1984;139(Pt 3):411–24.
10. Young BL, Begovac P, Stuart DG, et al. An effective sleeving technique in nerve repair. J Neurosci Methods 1984;10(1):51–8.
11. Madison RD, da Silva C, Dikkes P, et al. Peripheral nerve regeneration with entubulation repair: comparison of biodegradeable nerve guides versus polyethylene tubes and the effects of a laminin-containing gel. Exp Neurol 1987;95(2):378–90.
12. Henry EW, Chiu TH, Nyilas E, et al. Nerve regeneration through biodegradable polyester tubes. Exp Neurol 1985;90(3):652–76.
13. Seckel BR, Chiu TH, Nyilas E, et al. Nerve regeneration through synthetic biodegradable nerve guides: regulation by the target organ. Plast Reconstr Surg 1984;74(2):173–81.
14. Evans Gb K, Widmer M, Gürlek A, et al. Tissue engineered conduits: the use of biodegradable poly-DL-lactic-co-glycolic acid (PLGA) scaffolds in peripheral nerve regeneration. Berlin (Germany): Springer; 1998.
15. Rodriguez FJ, Gomez N, Perego G, et al. Highly permeable polylactide-caprolactone nerve guides enhance peripheral nerve regeneration through long gaps. Biomaterials 1999;20(16):1489–500.
16. den Dunnen W, van der Lei B, Robinson PH, et al. Biological performance of a degradable poly(lactic acid-ε-caprolactone) nerve guide: influence of tube dimensions. J Biomed Mater Res A 1995;29:757–66.
17. Lundborg G, Dahlin LB, Danielsen N, et al. Nerve regeneration in silicone chambers: influence of gap length and of distal stump components. Exp Neurol 1982;76(2):361–75.
18. Williams LR, Longo FM, Powell HC, et al. Spatial-temporal progress of peripheral nerve regeneration within a silicone chamber: parameters for a bioassay. J Comp Neurol 1983;218(4):460–70.
19. Zhao Q, Dahlin LB, Kanje M, et al. Repair of the transected rat sciatic nerve: matrix formation within implanted silicone tubes. Restor Neurol Neurosci 1993;5:197–204.

20. Williams LR, Varon S. Modification of fibrin matrix formation in situ enhances nerve regeneration in silicone chambers. J Comp Neurol 1985;231(2): 209–20.

21. Jenq CB, Coggeshall RE. Nerve regeneration through holey silicone tubes. Brain Res 1985; 361(1–2):233–41.

22. Jenq CB, Coggeshall RE. Permeable tubes increase the length of the gap that regenerating axons can span. Brain Res 1987;408(1–2):239–42.

23. Vleggeert-Lankamp CL, de Ruiter GC, Wolfs JF, et al. Pores in synthetic nerve conduits are beneficial to regeneration. J Biomed Mater Res A 2007; 80(4):965–82.

24. Kim DH, Connolly SE, Zhao S, et al. Comparison of macropore, semipermeable, and nonpermeable collagen conduits in nerve repair. J Reconstr Microsurg 1993;9(6):415–20.

25. Jenq CB, Jenq LL, Coggeshall RE. Nerve regeneration changes with filters of different pore size. Exp Neurol 1987;97(3):662–71.

26. Aebischer P, Guenard V, Brace S. Peripheral nerve regeneration through blind-ended semipermeable guidance channels: effect of the molecular weight cutoff. J Neurosci 1989;9(10):3590–5.

27. Guenard V, Valentini RF, Aebischer P. Influence of surface texture of polymeric sheets on peripheral nerve regeneration in a two-compartment guidance system. Biomaterials 1991;12(2):259–63.

28. de Ruiter GC, Onyeneho IA, Liang ET, et al. Methods for in vitro characterization of multichannel nerve tubes. J Biomed Mater Res A 2008;84(3):643–51.

29. Belkas JS, Munro CA, Shoichet MS, et al. Peripheral nerve regeneration through a synthetic hydrogel nerve tube. Restor Neurol Neurosci 2005;23(1):19–29.

30. Midha R, Munro CA, Dalton PD, et al. Growth factor enhancement of peripheral nerve regeneration through a novel synthetic hydrogel tube. J Neurosurg 2003;99(3):555–65.

31. Vleggeert-Lankamp CL. The role of evaluation methods in the assessment of peripheral nerve regeneration through synthetic conduits: a systematic review. Laboratory investigation. J Neurosurg 2007; 107(6):1168–89.

32. den Dunnen WF, van der Lei B, Schakenraad JM, et al. Poly(DL-lactide-epsilon-caprolactone) nerve guides perform better than autologous nerve grafts. Microsurgery 1996;17(7):348–57.

33. Dellon AL, Mackinnon SE. An alternative to the classical nerve graft for the management of the short nerve gap. Plast Reconstr Surg 1988;82(5): 849–56.

34. Mackinnon SE, Dellon AL, O'Brien JP. Changes in nerve fiber numbers distal to a nerve repair in the rat sciatic nerve model. Muscle Nerve 1991; 14(11):1116–22.

35. Ansselin AD, Fink T, Davey DF. Peripheral nerve regeneration through nerve guides seeded with adult Schwann cells. Neuropathol Appl Neurobiol 1997; 23(5):387–98.

36. Kim DH, Connolly SE, Kline DG, et al. Labeled Schwann cell transplants versus sural nerve grafts in nerve repair. J Neurosurg 1994;80(2):254–60.

37. Guenard V, Kleitman N, Morrissey TK, et al. Syngeneic Schwann cells derived from adult nerves seeded in semipermeable guidance channels enhance peripheral nerve regeneration. J Neurosci 1992;12(9):3310–20.

38. de Ruiter GC, Spinner RJ, Malessy MJA, et al, Accuracy of motor axon regeneration across autograft, single lumen, and multichannel poly(lactic-co-glycolic acid) (PLGA) nerve tubes. Neurosurgery 2008;63(1):144–53.

39. Valero-Cabre A, Tsironis K, Skouras E, et al. Superior muscle reinnervation after autologous nerve graft or poly-L-lactide-epsilon-caprolactone (PLC) tube implantation in comparison to silicone tube repair. J Neurosci Res 2001;63(2): 214–23.

40. Bodine-Fowler SC, Meyer RS, Moskovitz A, et al. Inaccurate projection of rat soleus motoneurons: a comparison of nerve repair techniques. Muscle Nerve 1997;20(1):29–37.

41. Evans PJ, Bain JR, Mackinnon SE, et al. Selective reinnervation: a comparison of recovery following microsuture and conduit nerve repair. Brain Res 1991;559(2):315–21.

42. Rende M, Granato A, Lo Monaco M, et al. Accuracy of reinnervation by peripheral nerve axons regenerating across a 10-mm gap within an impermeable chamber. Exp Neurol 1991;111(3):332–9.

43. Zhao Q, Dahlin LB, Kanje M, et al. Specificity of muscle reinnervation following repair of the transected sciatic nerve. A comparative study of different repair techniques in the rat. J Hand Surg [Br] 1992;17(3):257–61.

44. Brushart TM, Mathur V, Sood R, et al. Boyes Award. Dispersion of regenerating axons across enclosed neural gaps. J Biomed Mater Res A 1995;20(4):557–64.

45. Vleggeert-Lankamp CL, de Ruiter GC, Wolfs JF, et al. Type grouping in skeletal muscles after experimental reinnervation: another explanation. Eur J Neurosci 2005;21(5):1249–56.

46. de Medinaceli L, Freed WJ, Wyatt RJ. An index of the functional condition of rat sciatic nerve based on measurements made from walking tracks. Exp Neurol 1982;77:634–43.

47. Bain JR, Mackinnon SE, Hunter DA. Functional evaluation of complete sciatic, peroneal, and posterior tibial nerve lesions in the rat. Plast Reconstr Surg 1989;83(1):129–38.

48. Dellon AL, Mackinnon SE. Sciatic nerve regeneration in the rat. Validity of walking track assessment

in the presence of chronic contractures. Microsurgery 1989;10(3):220–5.

49. Weber RA, Proctor WH, Warner MR, et al. Autotomy and the sciatic functional index. Microsurgery 1993;14(5):323–7.

50. Fu SY, Gordon T. Contributing factors to poor functional recovery after delayed nerve repair: prolonged denervation. J Neurosci 1995;15(5 Pt 2): 3886–95.

51. de Ruiter GC, Spinner RJ, Alaid AO, et al. Two-dimensional digital video ankle motion analysis for assessment of function in the rat sciatic nerve model. J Peripher Nerv Syst 2007;12(3):216–22.

52. Yannas IV, Hill BJ. Selection of biomaterials for peripheral nerve regeneration using data from the nerve chamber model. Biomaterials 2004;25(9):1593–600.

53. Archibald SJ, Krarup C, Shefner J, et al. A collagen-based nerve guide conduit for peripheral nerve repair: an electrophysiological study of nerve regeneration in rodents and nonhuman primates. J Comp Neurol 1991;306(4):685–96.

54. Archibald SJ, Shefner J, Krarup C, et al. Monkey median nerve repaired by nerve graft or collagen nerve guide tube. J Neurosci 1995;15(5 Pt 2): 4109–23.

55. Mackinnon SE, Dellon AL. A study of nerve regeneration across synthetic (Maxon) and biologic (collagen) nerve conduits for nerve gaps up to 5 cm in the primate. J Reconstr Microsurg 1990;6(2):117–21.

56. Schlosshauer B, Dreesmann L, Schaller HE, et al. Synthetic nerve guide implants in humans: a comprehensive survey. Neurosurgery 2006;59(4): 740–7 [discussion: 747–8].

57. Stanec S, Stanec Z. Reconstruction of upper-extremity peripheral-nerve injuries with ePTFE conduits. J Reconstr Microsurg 1998;14(4):227–32.

58. Pitta MC, Wolford LM, Mehra P, et al. Use of Gore-Tex tubing as a conduit for inferior alveolar and lingual nerve repair: experience with 6 cases. J Oral Maxillofac Surg 2001;59(5):493–6 [discussion: 497].

59. Pogrel MA, McDonald AR, Kaban LB. Gore-Tex tubing as a conduit for repair of lingual and inferior alveolar nerve continuity defects: a preliminary report. J Oral Maxillofac Surg 1998;56(3):319–21 [discussion: 321–12].

60. Ashley WW Jr, Weatherly T, Park TS. Collagen nerve guides for surgical repair of brachial plexus birth injury. J Neurosurg 2006;105(6 Suppl):452–6.

61. Crawley WA, Dellon AL. Inferior alveolar nerve reconstruction with a polyglycolic acid bioabsorbable nerve conduit. Plast Reconstr Surg 1992; 90(2):300–2.

62. Kim J, Dellon AL. Reconstruction of a painful post-traumatic medial plantar neuroma with a bioabsorbable nerve conduit: a case report. J Foot Ankle Surg 2001;40(5):318–23.

63. Navissano M, Malan F, Carnino R, et al. Neurotube for facial nerve repair. Microsurgery 2005;25(4): 268–71.

64. Ducic I, Maloney CT Jr, Dellon AL. Reconstruction of the spinal accessory nerve with autograft or neurotube? Two case reports. J Reconstr Microsurg 2005;21(1):29–33 [discussion: 34].

65. Dellon AL, Maloney CT Jr. Salvage of sensation in a hallux-to-thumb transfer by nerve tube reconstruction. J Hand Surg [Am] 2006;31(9):1495–8.

66. Donoghoe N, Rosson GD, Dellon AL. Reconstruction of the human median nerve in the forearm with the Neurotube. Microsurgery 2007;27(7): 595–600.

67. Inada Y, Hosoi H, Yamashita A, et al. Regeneration of peripheral motor nerve gaps with a polyglycolic acid-collagen tube: technical case report. Neurosurgery 2007;61(5):E1105–7 [discussion: E1107].

68. Inada Y, Morimoto S, Takakura Y, et al. Regeneration of peripheral nerve gaps with a polyglycolic acid-collagen tube. Neurosurgery 2004;55(3): 640–6 [discussion: 646–8].

69. Hung V, Dellon AL. Reconstruction of a 4-cm human median nerve gap by including an autogenous nerve slice in a bioabsorbable nerve conduit: case report. J Hand Surg [Am] 2008; 33(3):313–5.

70. Fan W, Gu J, Hu W, et al. Repairing a 35-mm-long median nerve defect with a chitosan/PGA artificial nerve graft in the human: a case study. Microsurgery 2008;28(4):238–42.

71. Lundborg G, Rosen B, Dahlin L, et al. Tubular versus conventional repair of median and ulnar nerves in the human forearm: early results from a prospective, randomized, clinical study. J Hand Surg [Am] 1997;22(1):99–106.

72. Lundborg G, Rosen B, Dahlin L, et al. Tubular repair of the median or ulnar nerve in the human forearm: a 5-year follow-up. J Hand Surg [Br] 2004; 29(2):100–7.

73. Dellon AL. Use of a silicone tube for the reconstruction of a nerve injury. J Hand Surg [Br] 1994;19(3):271–2.

74. Meek MF, Coert JH, Hermens RA, et al. The use of silicone tubing in the late repair of the median and ulnar nerves in the forearm. J Hand Surg [Br] 2000; 25(4):408–9.

75. Merle M, Dellon AL, Campbell JN, et al. Complications from silicon-polymer intubulation of nerves. Microsurgery 1989;10(2):130–3.

76. Braga-Silva J. The use of silicone tubing in the late repair of the median and ulnar nerves in the forearm. J Hand Surg [Br] 1999;24(6):703–6.

77. Dahlin LB, Anagnostaki L, Lundborg G. Tissue response to silicone tubes used to repair human median and ulnar nerves. Scand J Plast Reconstr Surg Hand Surg 2001;35(1):29–34.

78. Dahlin L, Lundborg G. The use of silicone tubing in the late repair of the median and ulnar nerves in the forearm. J Hand Surg [Br] 2001;26(4):393–4.

79. Weber RA, Breidenbach WC, Brown RE, et al. A randomized prospective study of polyglycolic acid conduits for digital nerve reconstruction in humans. Plast Reconstr Surg 2000;106(5):1036–45 [discussion: 1046–8].

80. Mackinnon SE, Dellon AL. Clinical nerve reconstruction with a bioabsorbable polyglycolic acid tube. Plast Reconstr Surg 1990;85(3):419–24.

81. Moberg E. Two-point discrimination test. A valuable part of hand surgical rehabilitation, e.g. in tetraplegia. Scand J Rehabil Med 1990;22(3):127–34.

82. Battiston B, Geuna S, Ferrero M, et al. Nerve repair by means of tubulization: literature review and personal clinical experience comparing biological and synthetic conduits for sensory nerve repair. Microsurgery 2005;25(4):258–67.

83. Bertleff MJ, Meek MF, Nicolai JP. A prospective clinical evaluation of biodegradable Neurolac nerve guides for sensory nerve repair in the hand. J Hand Surg [Am] 2005;30(3):513–8.

84. Dellon ES, Keller KM, Moratz V, et al. Validation of cutaneous pressure threshold measurements for the evaluation of hand function. Ann Plast Surg 1997;38(5):485–92.

85. Meek MF, Coert JH. US Food and Drug Administration/Conformit Europe-approved absorbable nerve conduits for clinical repair of peripheral and cranial nerves. Ann Plast Surg 2008;60(1):110–6.

86. Madison RD, Da Silva CF, Dikkes P. Entubulation repair with protein additives increases the maximum nerve gap distance successfully bridged with tubular prostheses. Brain Res 1988;447(2):325–34.

87. Labrador RO, Buti M, Navarro X. Influence of collagen and laminin gels concentration on nerve regeneration after resection and tube repair. Exp Neurol 1998;149(1):243–52.

88. Valentini RF, Aebischer P, Winn SR, et al. Collagen- and laminin-containing gels impede peripheral nerve regeneration through semipermeable nerve guidance channels. Exp Neurol 1987;98(2):350–6.

89. Verdu E, Labrador RO, Rodriguez FJ, et al. Alignment of collagen and laminin-containing gels improve nerve regeneration within silicone tubes. Restor Neurol Neurosci 2002;20(5):169–79.

90. Rodriguez FJ, Verdu E, Ceballos D, et al. Nerve guides seeded with autologous Schwann cells improve nerve regeneration. Exp Neurol 2000;161(2):571–84.

91. Sinis N, Schaller HE, Schulte-Eversum C, et al. Nerve regeneration across a 2-cm gap in the rat median nerve using a resorbable nerve conduit filled with Schwann cells. J Neurosurg 2005; 103(6):1067–76.

92. Luo Y, Shoichet MS. A photolabile hydrogel for guided three-dimensional cell growth and migration. Nat Mater 2004;3(4):249–53.

93. Lundborg G, Dahlin L, Dohi D, et al. A new type of "bioartificial" nerve graft for bridging extended defects in nerves. J Hand Surg [Br] 1997;22(3): 299–303.

94. Matsumoto K, Ohnishi K, Kiyotani T, et al. Peripheral nerve regeneration across an 80-mm gap bridged by a polyglycolic acid (PGA)-collagen tube filled with laminin-coated collagen fibers: a histological and electrophysiological evaluation of regenerated nerves. Brain Res 2000;868(2): 315–28.

95. Wang X, Hu W, Cao Y, et al. Dog sciatic nerve regeneration across a 30-mm defect bridged by a chitosan/PGA artificial nerve graft. Brain 2005; 128(Pt 8):1897–910.

96. Nakamura T, Inada Y, Fukuda S, et al. Experimental study on the regeneration of peripheral nerve gaps through a polyglycolic acid-collagen (PGA-collagen) tube. Brain Res 2004;1027(1–2):18–29.

97. Francel PC, Francel TJ, Mackinnon SE, et al. Enhancing nerve regeneration across a silicone tube conduit by using interposed short-segment nerve grafts. J Neurosurg 1997;87(6):887–92.

98. Meek MF, Den Dunnen WF, Schakenraad JM, et al. Evaluation of functional nerve recovery after reconstruction with a poly (DL-lactide-epsilon-caprolactone) nerve guide, filled with modified denatured muscle tissue. Microsurgery 1996;17(10):555–61.

99. Yoshii S, Oka M. Peripheral nerve regeneration along collagen filaments. Brain Res 2001;888(1): 158–62.

100. Yoshii S, Oka M, Shima M, et al. Bridging a 30-mm nerve defect using collagen filaments. J Biomed Mater Res 2003;67A(2):467–74.

101. Sundback C, Hadlock T, Cheney M, et al. Manufacture of porous polymer nerve conduits by a novel low-pressure injection molding process. Biomaterials 2003;24(5):819–30.

102. Hadlock T, Sundback C, Hunter D, et al. A polymer foam conduit seeded with Schwann cells promotes guided peripheral nerve regeneration. Tissue Eng 2000;6(2):119–27.

103. Bender MD, Bennett JM, Waddell RL, et al. Multichanneled biodegradable polymer/CultiSpher composite nerve guides. Biomaterials 2004; 25(7-8):1269–78.

104. Yang Y, De Laporte L, Rives CB, et al. Neurotrophin releasing single and multiple lumen nerve conduits. J Control Release 2005;104(3):433–46.

105. Sinis N, Schaller HE, Becker ST, et al. Long nerve gaps limit the regenerative potential of bioartificial nerve conduits filled with Schwann cells. Restor Neurol Neurosci 2007;25(2):131–41.

106. Evans GR, Brandt K, Katz S, et al. Bioactive poly(L-lactic acid) conduits seeded with Schwann cells for peripheral nerve regeneration. Biomaterials 2002; 23(3):841–8.

107. Mimura T, Dezawa M, Kanno H, et al. Peripheral nerve regeneration by transplantation of bone marrow stromal cell-derived Schwann cells in adult rats. J Neurosurg 2004;101(5):806–12.

108. Rich KM, Alexander TD, Pryor JC, et al. Nerve growth factor enhances regeneration through silicone chambers. Exp Neurol 1989;105(2):162–70.

109. Whitworth IH, Brown RA, Dore CJ, et al. Nerve growth factor enhances nerve regeneration through fibronectin grafts. J Hand Surg [Br] 1996; 21(4):514–22.

110. Sterne GD, Brown RA, Green CJ, et al. Neurotrophin-3 delivered locally via fibronectin mats enhances peripheral nerve regeneration. Eur J Neurosci 1997;9(7):1388–96.

111. Santos X, Rodrigo J, Hontanilla B, et al. Evaluation of peripheral nerve regeneration by nerve growth factor locally administered with a novel system. J Neurosci Methods 1998;85(1):119–27.

112. Goraltchouk A, Scanga V, Morshead CM, et al. Incorporation of protein-eluting microspheres into biodegradable nerve guidance channels for controlled release. J Control Release 2006;110(2): 400–7.

113. Piotrowicz A, Shoichet MS. Nerve guidance channels as drug delivery vehicles. Biomaterials 2006; 27(9):2018–27.

114. Aebischer P, Valentini RF, Dario P, et al. Piezoelectric guidance channels enhance regeneration in the mouse sciatic nerve after axotomy. Brain Res 1987;436(1):165–8.

115. Schmidt CE, Shastri VR, Vacanti JP, et al. Stimulation of neurite outgrowth using an electrically conducting polymer. Proc Natl Acad Sci U S A 1997; 94(17):8948–53.

116. Li ST, Archibald SJ, Krarup C, et al. Peripheral nerve repair with collagen conduits. Clin Mater 1992;9(3–4):195–200.

117. Dalton PD, Flynn L, Shoichet MS. Manufacture of poly (2-hydroxyethyl methacrylate-co-methyl methacrylate) hydrogel tubes for use as nerve guidance channels. Biomaterials 2002;23:3843–51.

118. Evans GR, Brandt K, Widmer MS, et al. In vivo evaluation of poly(L-lactic acid) porous conduits for peripheral nerve regeneration. Biomaterials 1999; 20(12):1109–15.

119. Widmer MS, Gupta PK, Lu L, et al. Manufacture of porous biodegradable polymer conduits by an extrusion process for guided tissue regeneration. Biomaterials 1998;19(21):1945–55.

120. Perego G, Cella GD, Aldini NN, et al. Preparation of a new nerve guide from a poly(L-lactide-co-6-caprolactone). Biomaterials 1994;15(3):189–93.

121. den Dunnen WF, Meek MF, Grijpma DW, et al. In vivo and in vitro degradation of poly[(50)/(50) ((85)/(15) (L)/(D))LA/epsilon-CL], and the implications for the use in nerve reconstruction. J Biomed Mater Res 2000;51(4):575–85.

122. Meek MF, Van Der Werff JF, Nicolai JP, et al. Biodegradable p(DLLA-epsilon-CL) nerve guides versus autologous nerve grafts: electromyographic and video analysis. Muscle Nerve 2001;24(6):753–9.

123. Schappacher M, Fabre T, Mingotaud AF, et al. Study of a (trimethylenecarbonate-co-epsilon-caprolactone) polymer part 1: preparation of a new nerve guide through controlled random copolymerization using rare earth catalysts. Biomaterials 2001;22(21):2849–55.

124. Rosen B, Lundborg G. A model instrument for the documentation of outcome after nerve repair. J Hand Surg [Am] 2000;25(3):535–43.

From the Battlefront: Peripheral Nerve Surgery in Modern Day Warfare

James M. Ecklund, MD, FACS, COL (Ret), MC[a,b],*,
Geoffrey S.F. Ling, MD, COL, MC[c]

KEYWORDS

• Nerve injury • Gunshot wound • Prosthesis

Care of peripheral nerve injuries has been challenging military surgeons for centuries. British surgeons followed the nihilistic pattern of the times, recommending no treatment for divided nerves during the Napoleonic wars.[1] During the U.S. Civil War, Mitchell and colleagues[2] observed functional recovery of injured limbs but attributed it to the overlap from adjacent nerve innervations. In World War I, 3129 peripheral nerve injuries were recorded in the U.S. Armed Forces alone.[3] This incidence provided opportunities to compare several techniques of nerve repair, and many important conclusions on the repair of peripheral nerve injuries were published throughout the 1920s and 1930s.[4]

In World War II, 25,000 peripheral nerve injuries were evaluated by the Army Medical Corps. In 1944, a peripheral nerve registry was ordered by the Surgeon General of the U.S. Army; and in 1956, Woodhall and Beebe[5] published a study entitled "Peripheral Nerve Regeneration: A Follow-Up study of 3,656 World War II Injuries." The British also had a large experience with treating these injuries at multiple sites, including more than 2500 cases treated at Oxford.[6,7]

One of the largest modern series was published by clinicians at the Belgrade Military Medical Academy, where 3091 missile-induced peripheral nerve injuries were managed from 1991 to 1995. In several articles, Roganovic and colleagues[8–12] report functional outcomes on the repairs of 119 tibial,

157 peroneal, 128 ulnar, 81 median, and 131 radial nerves. The surgical results in the civilian population are also well categorized by several other experienced authors, including many large series by Dr. David Kline and colleagues.[13–21] The techniques for surgical management of blunt and sharp penetrating wounds in the military population are the same as those described for similar wounds in the civilian population.

Most military peripheral nerve injuries result from high-velocity gunshot wounds or fragments from explosions, resulting in blunt nerve injuries. Initial treatment is frequently performed by orthopedists or general surgeons, and attention is focused on stabilizing fractures, debriding necrotic tissue, repairing vascular damage, and preventing infection. Because of the extensive soft tissue damage frequently present, these wounds will often require multiple washouts. When identified, the status of injured nerves should be documented. Any nerve stumps should be tacked down to prevent retraction, and reconstructed in the ensuing weeks.

To guide surgical management, patients who have neuromas in continuity should be followed up clinically and elecrodiagnostically over the next several months to assess for evidence of spontaneous recovery. Indications, techniques with intraoperative nerve action potential recordings, and timing of exploration are well covered elsewhere, and do not differ from those presented in civilian

a Department of Neurosciences, Inova Fairfax Hospital, Falls Church, VA, USA
b Uniformed Services University, 4301 Jones Bridge Road, Bethesda, MD 20814, USA
c Neurology Department, Uniformed Services University, 4301 Jones Bridge Road, Bethesda, MD 20814, USA
* Corresponding author. Uniformed Services University, 4301 Jones Bridge Road, Bethesda, Maryland 20814.
E-mail address: james.ecklund@inova.org (J.M. Ecklund).

Neurosurg Clin N Am 20 (2009) 107–110
doi:10.1016/j.nec.2008.07.022
1042-3680/08/$ – see front matter © 2008 Elsevier Inc. All rights reserved.

literature. Also similar to the civilian literature, outcomes are related to the nerve and level of injury, timing of the repair, length of the nerve defect, and health of the surrounding tissue and vascular bed.

Pain is a common manifestation of peripheral nerve injury. A meta-analysis of the literature for "causalgia" published in 2003 found that high-velocity missile injuries accounted for 77% of reported cases.[22] In 2006, Roganovic and Mandic-Gajic[23,24] categorized missile-induced peripheral nerve injury into four different types of pain syndromes: deafferentation pain, neuropathic pain, complex regional pain syndrome type II (CRPS-II), and reinnervation pain. Of 2239 patients available for follow-up, 326 (14.6%) had a clinically significant pain syndrome; this represented 2652 (12.3%) of the prospectively assessed nerve injuries. Of these 326 patients, 258 (79.1%) underwent surgical exploration.

The United States and its allies have been treating casualties from the global war on terrorism since 2001. Since the onset of hostilities in October 2001 through January 2005, 1566 U.S. Service Members sustained 6609 combat wounds, according to the Joint Theater Trauma Registry. This figure does not include soldiers killed in action, returned to duty within 72 hours, or non–battle-related injuries. Distribution of these wounds included 29.4% head and neck, 5.6% thoracic, 10.7% abdominal, and 54.1% extremity. The extremity percentage is consistent with previous conflicts, whereas the head and neck percentage is higher. The mechanism of injury was 81% explosion and 19% gunshot, which varies from the historical explosion percentage of 65% to 73% between World War II and Vietnam.[25] The extremity injuries were evenly distributed between the upper and lower extremities: 129 (4%) were amputations, 915 (26%) were fractures, 1881 (53%) were soft tissue wounds, and 144 (4%) were nerve injuries.[26]

Publications reporting data from previous conflicts typically lag 10 to 20 years behind while data are collected, analyzed, and eventually published. Publications are sparse on peripheral nerve injuries from the current conflict (the War on Terrorism). This paucity can be explained by the relatively short interval since the onset of the conflict, the fact that the casualties are still being received, and the wide distribution of rehabilitative care at centers throughout the country, which impedes efficient follow-up data collection efforts. Publications are expected to emerge over the next 5 to 10 years, which will better evaluate the long-term results of current therapy and treatment strategies.

Approximately 90% of the casualties evacuated back to the United States from the global war on terrorism undergo their initial stateside treatment at either Walter Reed Army Medical Center or National Naval Medical Center. Before the conflict, a multidisciplinary peripheral nerve clinic, including orthopedics, physical medicine and rehabilitation, neurosurgery, and neurology, was established under the leadership of Dr. Neal Naff. This clinic still operates and has provided evaluation and treatment for a large number of casualties who had peripheral nerve injuries over the years. The number of patients who had any pain syndrome, including CRPS, has been extremely low. For the previously noted reasons, exact numbers are not yet tabulated and published; however, in the authors' 2-year experience in this clinic, only one surgical exploration was required to treat neuropathic pain.

This apparent reduction in missile-related casualties is commonly attributed to the aggressive early use of advanced regional anesthesia. Since 2003, Dr. Chip Buckenmier has championed the use of regional anesthesia in combat casualties.[27] Previously used in a limited form in Vietnam,[28] this technique calls for early intervention on the battlefield and during evacuation, using peripheral nerve blocks, continuous-infusion peripheral nerve catheters, and patient-controlled anesthesia when appropriate for patients who have injured limbs. These techniques have been used on 70% of combat amputees and 57% of a reported series of 500 battle-related extremity injuries that underwent surgery at Walter Reed Army Medical Center between March 2003 and December 2004.[29] Peripheral nerve catheter infusions are gradually tapered over several days to weeks, often transitioning to opiates, which are more gradually tapered. Tricyclic antidepressants, nonsteroidal anti-inflammatory medications, and anticonvulsants are also used liberally. Although more rigorous outcome data will need to be analyzed and published from this strategy, applying pain control with advanced regional anesthesia may markedly reduce the incidence of pain syndromes from blast- or missile-induced peripheral nerve injury.

Regardless of mechanism or location of a peripheral nerve injury, pain-free functional restoration remains the primary goal. The results of primary nerve grafting for motor and sensory functional restoration is well documented in many outstanding monographs, and remains dependent on the location of the injury, timing of the repair, and need for a graft. Much attention has recently focused on blast injury as it relates to traumatic brain injury, and research efforts are ongoing to better define the response of the brain to overpressure, electromagnetic pulse, and other less-studied components of a blast. No current clinical evidence suggests that peripheral nerve injuries sustained as a result of blast have a worse recovery potential than those sustained by a gunshot wound; however, it is an intriguing concept and may warrant further investigation.

Functional results of nerve repair procedures are often suboptimal. The Defense Advanced Research Program Agency has launched an extensive program designed to improve functional restoration for upper-extremity amputees that may have implications for peripheral nerve surgery in the future. This program has two components: development of a fully functional artificial upper extremity, and further development of the neural–machine interface to obtain complete integrated control of this advanced prosthesis. Amazing progress has been made in both areas. The current limb developed for the program has an 8-lb grip capability, 10-lb wrist capability, 20-lb elbow capability, 9° of freedom, receptors for 2-point discrimination up to 2 mm at the fingertips, pressure sensation at 0.25 N, temperature differentiation up to 10°F, and proprioceptive capability up to 10°. The next-generation arm will have 21° of freedom, full range of motion with proportional tactile receptors, and cosmetic appearance undifferentiated from human skin and form.

The neural–machine interface component of the project is more complex. Significant successes have already been reported with indirect neural control. At Northwestern University, Kuiken and colleagues[30] used a technique called *targeted reinnervation* to allow a patient who had high upper-extremity amputation to control a prosthetic limb. In this patient, neural transfers were performed from the ulnar, median, musculocutaneous, and radial nerves to motor nerves supplying different parts of the pectoralis major or serratus anterior. Two sensory branches were coapted end-to side into the median and ulnar nerves. Reenervation was allowed to occur and then computer analysis was used to translate muscle firing in the pectoralis region into artificial arm movement. Sensory feedback was provided by thumping the pectoralis, which had been reinnervated by ulnar and median afferents.[30]

Work is progressing in the development of electrode arrays for implantation into injured peripheral nerves above an injury site, where afferent and efferent impulses may be captured or delivered through wireless interaction with a distal robotic limb using computer technology. To accomplish truly fine dexterous control of finger movement, most researchers believe the interface will need to more directly connect with the motor and sensory cortex of the brain.

Early experiments have already provided proof of concept. A primate model has learned to perform simple tasks with a robotic arm using a direct cerebral cortex interface. More sophisticated work is ongoing for individual finger actuation using this type of neural–machine interface. The ultimate goal is the creation of a completely integrated, totally functional prosthetic limb. Although this research is being conducted with amputees in mind, these artificial limbs may eventually provide a functional restoration superior to what can be obtained with direct nerve repair techniques. This may eventually alter the approach to patients who have a severely impaired limb from peripheral nerve injury. If replacing affected limbs can provide more robust functional improvement with an acceptable complication profile, patients may choose amputation over direct nerve repair in some cases.

Throughout history, warfare has led to several medical advances. Management of peripheral nerve injury has similarly developed as a result of experience with treating combat wounds. The current conflict is also providing opportunities for medical refinements to improve the care and understanding of disease. The initial impression is that a reduced incidence of pain syndromes is present in casualties who have peripheral nerve injuries as a result of more aggressive early pain control using advanced regional anesthesia techniques, but long-term outcome studies must still be completed to validate this observation. Functional restoration using a new generation of advanced prosthetic devices may soon exceed that which can be obtained through biologic repair of nerve tissue.

REFERENCES

1. Guthrie JG. A treatise on gunshot wounds. London: C. Wood; 1827. p. 559.
2. Mitchell SW, Morehouse GR, Keen WW. Gunshot wounds and other injuries of nerves. Philadelphia: Lippincott; 1864. p. 377.
3. Frazier CH. Results of peripheral nerve surgery: incidence of peripheral nerve injuries. In: Weed FW, editor. The Medical Department of the United States Army in the World War. Vol 11, section 3. Washington, DC: US Government Printing Office; 1923. p. 749.
4. Naff NJ, Ecklund JM. History of peripheral nerve surgery techniques. Neurosurg Clin N Am 2001; 12(1):197–209.
5. Woodhall B, Beebe GW. Peripheral nerve regeneration: a follow-up study of 3,656 World War II injuries. Washington, DC: US Government Printing Office; 1956. p. xix.

6. Seddon HJ. The use of autogenous grafts for the repair of large gaps in peripheral nerves. Br J Surg 1964;33:317.

7. Seddon HJ. Peripheral nerve injuries in Great Britain during World War II: a review. Arch Neurol Psychiatry 1950;63:171–3.

8. Roganovic Z, Pavlicevic G, Petkovic S. Missle-induced complete lesions of the tibial nerve and tibial division of the sciatic nerve: results of 119 repairs. J Neurosurg 2005;103(4):622–9.

9. Roganovic Z. Missle-caused complete lesions of the peroneal nerve and peroneal division of the sciatic nerve: results of 157 repairs. J Neurosurg 2005; 57(6):1201–12 [discussion: 1201–212].

10. Roganovic Z. Missle-caused ulnar nerve injuries: outcomes of 128 repairs. Neurosurgery 2004;55(5): 1120–9.

11. Roganovic Z. Missle-caused median nerve injuries: results of 81 repairs. Surg Neurol 2005;63(5):410–8 [discussion: 418–19].

12. Roganovic Z, Petkovic S. Missile severences of the radial nerve: results of 131 repairs. Acta Neurochir(Wein) 2004;146(11):1185–92.

13. Kim DH, Murovic JA, Tiel RL, et al. Gunshot wounds involving the brachial plexus: surgical techniques and outcomes. J Reconstr Microsurg 2006;22(2): 67–72.

14. Kim DH, Murovic JA, Tiel RL, et al. Penetrating injuries due to gunshot wounds involving the brachial plexus. Neurosurg Focus 2004;16(5):E3 [review].

15. Kim DH, Murovic JA, Tiel RL, et al. Management and outcomes in 318 operative common peroneal nerve lesions at the Louisiana State University Health Sciences Center. Neurosurgery 2004;54(6):1421–8 [discussion: 1428–9].

16. Kim DH, Murovic JA, Tiel RL, et al. Surgical management and results of 135 tibial nerve lesions at the Louisiana State University Health Sciences Center. Neurosurgery 2003;53(5):1114–24 [discussion: 1124–5].

17. Kim DH, Cho YJ, Tiel RL, et al. Surgical outcomes of 111 spinal accessory nerve injuries. Neurosurgery 2003;53(5):1106–12 [discussion: 1102–3].

18. Kim DH, Han K, Tiel RL, et al. Surgical outcomes of 654 ulnar nerve injuries. J Neurosurg 2003;98(5): 993–1004.

19. Kim DH, Murovic JA, Tiel RL, et al. Management and outcomes of 42 surgical suprascapular nerve injuries and entrapments. Neurosurgery 2005; 57(1):120–7 [discussion: 120–7].

20. Kim DH, Murovic JA, Tiel RL, et al. Management and outcomes in 353 surgically treated sciatic nerve lesions. J Neurosurg 2004;101(1):8–17.

21. Kim DH, Murovic JA, Tiel RL, et al. Intrapelvic and thigh-level femoral nerve lesions: management and outcomes in 119 surgically treated cases. J Neurosurg 2004;100(6):989–96.

22. Hassantash SA, Afrakhteh M, Maier RV. Causalgia: a meta-analysis of the Literature. Arch Surg 2003; 138:1226–31.

23. Roganovic Z, Mandic-Gajic G. Pain syndromes after missile-caused peripheral nerve lesions: part 1-clinical characteristics. Neurosurgery 2006;59(6): 1226–37.

24. Roganovic Z, Mandic-Gajic G. Pain syndromes after missile-caused peripheral nerve lesions: part 2-Treatment. Neurosurgery 2006;59(6):1238–51.

25. Owens BD, Kragh JF, Wenke JC, et al. Combat wounds in operation Iraqi freedom and operation enduring freedom. J Trauma 2008;64:295–9.

26. Owens BD, Kragh JF, Macaitis J, et al. Characterization of extremity wounds in operation Iraqi freedom and operation enduring freedom. J Orthop Trauma 2007;21(4):254–7.

27. Hampton T. Researchers probe nerve-blocking pain treatment for wounded soldiers. JAMA 2007; 297(22):2461–2.

28. Thompson GE. Narration: anesthesia for battle casualties in Vietnam. JAMA 1967;201:218–9.

29. Stojadinovic A, Auton A, Peoples GE, et al. Responding to challenges in modern combat casualty care: innovative use of advanced regional anesthesia. Pain Med 2006;7(4):330–8.

30. Kuiken T, Miller L, Lipschutz RD, et al. Targeted reinnervation for enhanced prosthetic arm function in a woman with a proximal amputation: a case study. Lancet 2007;369:371–80.

Neurostimulation Techniques for Painful Peripheral Nerve Disorders

R. Morgan Stuart, MD, Christopher J. Winfree, MD, FACS*

KEYWORDS

- Extraforaminal spinal nerve root stimulation
- Intraspinal nerve root stimulation • Pain
- Peripheral nerve field stimulation
- Peripheral nerve stimulation
- Spinal nerve root stimulation
- Subcutaneous peripheral nerve stimulation
- Transforaminal spinal nerve root stimulation
- Trans-spinal nerve root stimulation

The problem of pain in peripheral nerve injuries has presented a unique challenge to physicians throughout history. From Mitchell's earliest descriptions of causalgia in the 1800s,[1] the treatment of pain in peripheral nerve injuries has involved the work of clinicians, neurologists, psychiatrists, anesthesiologists, and surgeons. The pain of peripheral nerve injuries is often unremitting and agonizing, causing significant physical and psychologic disability in these patients. Furthermore, without adequate treatment, this pain and suffering can be expected to continue throughout life, preventing the patient from working or performing many activities of daily living. Many treatments and treatment modalities have been developed through the years to treat these pains, such as opiates, anticonvulsants, antidepressants, and physical and psychologic therapies, but for some patients these provide inadequate relief from their pain.

The gate control theory of pain, proposed in the 1960s, suggested that altering the function of certain sensory pathways in the spinal cord could attenuate the subjective experience of pain by attenuating the activity in separate but parallel pain pathways.[2] Soon thereafter, the first applications of this concept appeared in people. Neuromodulation, the therapeutic alteration of activity in pain pathways with the use of an implantable device, was reported in 1967 as both peripheral nerve stimulation (PNS)[3] and spinal cord stimulation (SCS).[4] The former enabled the targeting of stimulation paresthesias and subsequent pain relief within a specific peripheral nerve distribution, whereas the latter permitted more regional areas of coverage, such as the lower extremities.

Although the process of neuromodulation still is not understood completely, it is thought to involve both inhibition and activation of relevant neural circuitry, including pain pathways in the dorsal horn nucleus and the autonomic nervous system.[5] More recent studies have elucidated the role of neurotransmitters such as g-aminobutyric acid and adenosine to explain how pain modulation through neurostimulation is accomplished.[5] The success of SCS has been documented in several randomized–control trials and case series[6–9] and has provided the impetus for the development of various techniques to target pain control by applying electrical current to different sensory pathways along the peripheral nervous system. The technique of stimulation along a specific spinal nerve

Department of Neurological Surgery, Columbia University Medical Center, 710 West 168th Street, New York, NY 10032, USA
* Corresponding author.
E-mail address: cjw12@columbia.edu (C.J. Winfree).

Neurosurg Clin N Am 20 (2009) 111–120
doi:10.1016/j.nec.2008.07.027
1042-3680/08/$ – see front matter © 2008 Elsevier Inc. All rights reserved.

neurosurgery.theclinics.com

root or roots, called spinal nerve root stimulation (SNRS),[10,11] offers the advantages of both SCS and PNS. There are also some pain syndromes that are either not amenable to or are served incompletely by SCS, PNS, or SNRS and for which the technique of subcutaneous peripheral nerve stimulation (SPNS) has emerged. All of these techniques are built on a basic set of underlying principles and techniques for implantation, with a common goal of accurately targeting and treating neuropathic pain while at the same time minimizing unwanted adverse effects. Now, within the context of a comprehensive, multidisciplinary approach to pain management, these neurostimulation techniques may offer hope to those patients for whom pain relief was previously unattainable.

SPINAL CORD STIMULATION
Description

Since its introduction over 40 years ago, SCS has undergone significant advancements in technology and techniques for placement. Although the mechanisms by which electrical stimulation of the dorsal columns and afferent fibers attenuate or modulate a patient's sensation of pain are not understood completely, their efficacy in practice has been established, and SCS techniques have been described in the literature for decades.[5] In general, SCS consists of placing an electrode array in the epidural space along the posterior aspect of the dorsal columns. Any point along the spinal cord is a potential target, but generally, midcervical cord placement allows for upper extremity coverage; lower thoracic cord placement allows for low back and lower extremity coverage, and midthoracic cord placement allows for abdominal and visceral coverage.[12] Individual electrode arrays may be placed over each hemicord, allowing for the independent control of left and right sides separately.

Indications

SCS remains the most commonly used implantable neurostimulation technique for the management of a growing number of pain syndromes and regional pain problems. These include: radiculopathies, failed back surgery syndrome (FBSS), peripheral neuropathy, peripheral vascular disease, chronic unstable angina, pain of spinal origin, and complex regional pain syndrome.[5] It generally is accepted for all types of neurostimulation that if a patient has a surgical option with a good probability of success in providing relief for his or her pain (other than SCS), as in the case of a radiculopathy that correlates anatomically with a herniated lumbar disc on MRI, that the patient undergo the definitive surgical procedure rather than treatment with an implantable device. And although SCS implantation is a relatively safe procedure, less invasive alternatives should be used first, before a patient is recommended for SCS. Formal psychologic evaluation generally is recommended before implantation to rule out psychologic amplifiers of pain.

Technique

A trial of SCS is performed before permanent implantation. The trial involves percutaneous placement of a single, or multiple if necessary, cylindric electrode lead(s) percutaneously under conscious sedation using fluoroscopic guidance. An interlaminar space several levels below the level of desired stimulation is selected, and a spinal needle inserted off the midline to access the epidural space. The electrode then is threaded up to the desired spinal level under fluoroscopic guidance. The exact lead position depends upon the desired pattern of stimulation. For example, midline placement of the electrode generally gives bilateral stimulation paresthesias, whereas lateral placement provides unilateral coverage. The leads then are connected to an external stimulus generator, and the patient reports subjective response to stimulation. The leads may be repositioned to achieve optimal coverage. The patient is discharged home for a trial of stimulation of 1 week in most cases. If the response is favorable, the patient returns for permanent implantation of the electrodes and the implantable pulse generator. For permanent placement, either percutaneous or paddle-type electrodes are used, with the latter used predominantly to minimize the risk of migration. Placement of the paddle electrode requires a small minilaminectomy to be performed, under conscious sedation or general anesthesia. The leads are anchored to the fascia to minimize the risk of migration. The leads then are tunneled to a subcutaneous implantable pulse generator (**Fig. 1**).

Limitations

Electrical stimulation of the spinal cord has some limitations. Lead migration, progressive loss of efficacy over time, and postural variability in stimulation intensity (related to the mobility of the spinal cord within the spinal canal during patient movement) are all examples of potential problems with these systems.[5] In addition, SCS provides incomplete or inconsistent coverage of many areas, which are often problem areas for patients who have chronic pain, including the low back, buttocks, feet, groin, pelvis, and neck.[10] Furthermore, some pathways such as those supplying the S2–5 dermatomes, are located somatotopically deep within the spinal cord, and tend to be out of reach

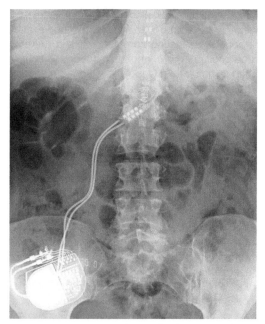

Fig. 1. Anteroposterior radiograph of a patient following placement of a spinal cord stimulator at a low thoracic level and an implantable pulse generator in the buttock to treat complex regional pain syndrome of the lower extremity.

from SCS. Pain syndromes located in these areas are often more responsive to other forms of neurostimulation.

PERIPHERAL NERVE STIMULATION
Description

Disorders of the peripheral nervous system often present a unique challenge to the clinician or surgeon, because the neuropathic pain associated with them can be extremely resistant to typical pain treatments. Painful peripheral nerve disorders often have pain in a particular peripheral nerve distribution, and thus an optimal treatment modality is one that delivers targeted relief to the precise distribution of the pain. This represents the primary advantage of PNS—the ability to focus stimulation paresthesias into the distribution of a specific peripheral nerve without providing unwanted stimulation into other areas. To that end, PNS has undergone several refinements in recent years, enabling the treatment of painful peripheral nerve problems that until fairly recently were either untreatable or poorly treated with traditional SCS techniques.

Indications

Generally speaking, PNS is indicated when the pain is confined to the distribution of a single peripheral nerve, or a limited number of individual

peripheral nerves. It is also important that placing the electrode array along the desired peripheral nerve can be done at least as easily as other forms of neurostimulation that also could treat the pain syndrome reasonably. For example, it makes little sense to perform a substantial sciatic nerve exploration at a buttock level to place PNS electrodes, when a spinal cord stimulator could achieve similar pattern of coverage much less invasively.

As techniques for preferentially stimulating the peripheral nervous system have evolved, so too has the spectrum of pathology amenable to treatment by these novel techniques. The use of PNS to treat craniofacial neuropathic pain has emerged in the last decade as a viable treatment modality for this disorder. Because SCS is, for the most part, ineffective in treating craniofacial pain, PNS marks an exiting new therapeutic alternative for patients suffering from a wide array of craniofacial pain syndromes. It most commonly is used to stimulate the occipital and trigeminal regions, for various conditions affecting these nerve distributions. The use of this technique has been reported in the literature to treat postherpetic neuralgia involving the supraorbital and infraorbital nerves,[13–18] as well as occipital nerve[19–22] dysfunction following trauma or surgery, atypical migraines presenting with occipital pain,[23,24] cluster headache,[25] and cervicogenic occipital pain.[23,24,26–28] PNS also may be used to target larger nerves through an open approach.[27] For example, tibial and peroneal nerve stimulation may provide relief of foot pain.

Technique

As with SCS implantation, rigorous methodology for patient selection, including consideration of alternative, less invasive pharmacologic, physical medicine, or psychologic therapies should be applied to ensure the greatest success with peripheral nerve stimulator implantation. Similar to SCS, the same basic paradigm exists for PNS placement anywhere in the body. Following psychologic evaluation, a trial of stimulation is performed. Although not routinely done at the authors' institution, a diagnostic nerve block commonly is performed initially to establish the peripheral nerve contribution to the pain.[23,24]

For percutaneous PNS, electrodes are inserted in the epifascial plane above the muscle under conscious sedation. Four- or eight-contact electrodes are used, depending upon the desired size of electrode array. For craniofacial stimulation, fluoroscopic guidance typically is not required, as the external facial landmarks are adequate for guidance, although it may be used to verify positioning and make fine tune adjustments if coverage is inadequate. For stimulation of the supraorbital nerve, the standard landmarks for insertion are the supraorbital groove or foramen and the supraorbital ridge. For the infraorbital nerve, the infraorbital foramen and the floor of the orbit are used (**Fig. 2**). For the occipital nerve, our entry point is on midline near the occipital protuberance. The curved needle is advanced in a superolateral direction, aiming for the top of the pinna. Thus, the octad electrode overlies the occipital nerves (**Fig. 3**). Following placement, the electrode is connected to an external pulse generator and the patient tested for stimulation-induced paresthesias. Coverage areas also are tested. If the result is satisfactory, the electrode leads are fastened to the skin in a looped fashion with a series of 3-0 silk ties to avoid excessive strain or torque on the electrodes. An anteroposterior and lateral skull radiograph are obtained to document the electrode placement, and the patient then is discharged home for a trial of stimulation of typically 1 week. The authors do not prescribe antibiotic prophylaxis routinely for the trial duration. If the trial provides a distinct benefit, the patient returns for replacement of the temporary electrode with a permanent one. A new electrode then is tunneled to an implantable pulse generator, which is placed subcutaneously in either a buttock or subclavicular location.

For open PNS, the target peripheral nerve is subjected to an external neurolysis with the patient under conscious sedation. Then either a percutaneous or paddle lead is placed adjacent to the nerve (**Fig. 4**). When using a paddle lead, the authors customarily place a layer of fascia between the electrode array and the nerve itself. Intraoperative testing commences, and the electrode positioned is changed as needed to achieve optimal stimulation. Once in position, it is secured with sutures to surrounding tissue planes, and externalized with a disposable extension wire. After wound closure, the patient undergoes a 1-week trial as for the percutaneous system. If successful, the extension wire is discarded, and the lead connected to a nearby implantable pulse generator as described previously. If the trial was unhelpful, the lead is removed and discarded.

Limitations

The primary drawback to PNS is lead migration and fracture. Although spinal cord stimulators are placed along the relatively stable and immobile spine, PNS requires sometimes difficult surgical access to the target nerves, which are often in regions of the body such as the neck or extremities that are highly mobile, placing high levels of stress along the course of the electrode system and theoretically contributing to higher rates of electrode migration and malfunction. And while the selective stimulation of a single peripheral nerve may be desired, in cases where broader coverage of a particular area of pain distribution is necessary, a single peripheral nerve stimulator alone may be inadequate.

SPINAL NERVE ROOT STIMULATION
Description

One of the more recent and exciting developments in neurostimulation involves the preferential stimulation of one or more spinal nerve roots directly. Thus, desired stimulation can be targeted to specific radicular distributions while eliminating unwanted paresthesias beyond these specific areas. Numerous electrode placement strategies have been developed to selectively stimulate spinal nerve roots, and previously have been classified to include the intraspinal (anterograde or retrograde), transforaminal, trans-spinal, and extraforaminal techniques.[11] Like SCS, these stimulators are located along the relatively stable and immobile spine, theoretically limiting the risk of electrode migration compared with more peripherally-placed PNS electrodes.

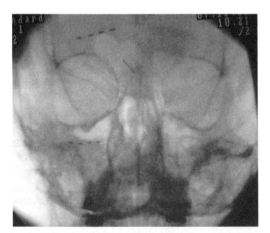

Fig. 2. Anteroposterior radiograph of a patient following placement of supraorbital and infraorbital nerve stimulator electrodes to treat trigeminal neuropathic pain resulting from a trigeminal branch injury. Note the position of the electrodes in the vicinity of the nerves as they exit their respective foramina near the orbit.

Indications

Intraspinal nerve root stimulation has become a useful technique for treating painful peripheral nerve problems. In this form of SNRS, the electrode is placed in the lateral aspect of the spinal

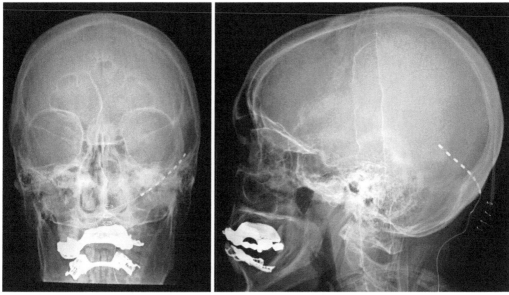

Fig. 3. Anteroposterior (*left*) and lateral (*right*) radiographs of a patient following placement of an occipital nerve stimulator electrode used to treat occipital neuralgia. The electrode array overlies the occipital nerves as they course along the back of the head. Either percutaneous or paddle leads may be used in this location.

canal, overlying the desired dorsal rootlets. In this fashion, stimulation paresthesias are focused along the target nerve root dermatomes, and not along more caudal targets as in dorsal column stimulation. Postherniorrhaphy inguinal neuralgias may be treated with an intraspinal nerve root electrode placed in the lateral spinal canal at the T12-L1 level eccentric to the side of pain (**Fig. 5**). This focuses stimulation paresthesias in the groin region without annoying lower extremity stimulation. The intraspinal retrograde approach has

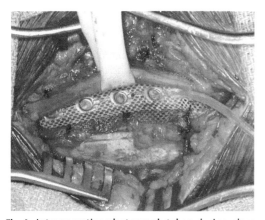

Fig. 4. Intraoperative photograph taken during placement of a tibial nerve stimulator following external neurolysis of the nerve. Although a paddle electrode was used to treat tibial neuralgia in this case, percutaneous electrodes may be used also.

demonstrated applicability in treating pelvic pain,[29] perineal pain of urologic origin,[30] and interstitial cystitis.[31–33]

Transforaminal nerve root stimulation is a form of SNRS in which the electrodes are passed through the spinal canal in a retrograde fashion, and steered out into the nerve root foramen. Once in place, the stimulation paresthesias are focused upon the single nerve root and its dorsal root ganglion residing in the target foramen. Although traditional SCS covers the dorsal columns only, stimulating pathways mediating touch, vibration, and proprioception, stimulation of the dorsal root ganglion theoretically applies additional current to spinothalamic tracts mediating temperature sensation.[34,35] Thus, neuropathic pain syndromes that feature predominantly deranged temperature sensation may be served uniquely by the transforaminal technique. Successful transforaminal nerve root stimulation has been reported in patients who have ilioinguinal neuralgia,[36] discogenic back pain,[30] FBSS,[37] and interstitial cystitis.[31–33] The authors have used transforaminal nerve root stimulation to treat foot pain from painful peripheral neuropathy (**Fig. 6**), a notoriously difficult peripheral nerve pain disorder to treat.

Technique

Intraspinal nerve root stimulation can be accomplished through either an anterograde or

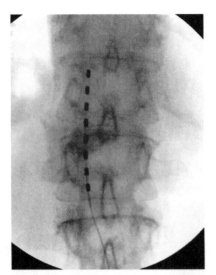

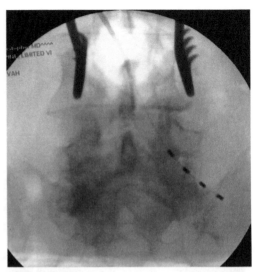

Fig. 5. Intraoperative fluoroscopic image of a patient during placement of a right-sided intraspinal nerve root electrode at the T12-L1 level used to treat postherpetic neuralgia at a groin level. Note the placement of the electrode in the lateral aspect of the spinal canal, overlying the dorsal rootlets before their entry into the dorsal root entry zone. This focuses the stimulation paresthesias into the T12-L1 dermatomes selectively without unwanted stimulation into the dorsal columns or other nerve roots. The authors commonly use this same electrode array to treat postherniorrhaphy inguinal neuralgias when less invasive measures are unhelpful.

Fig. 6. Intraoperative fluoroscopic image of a patient during placement of a left-sided transforaminal nerve root electrode at the L5 level used to treat a painful peripheral neuropathy. The L5 nerve root was chosen, because the patient's pain was concentrated along the top of his foot. Note placement of the electrode within the neural foramen, in a position overlying both the spinal nerve root and the dorsal root ganglion.

retrograde percutaneous approach. In this technique, the electrode is located completely within the spinal canal. In the retrograde approach, the introducer needle is directed into the epidural space and the electrode passed in a retrograde and lateral fashion parallel to and overlying the desired nerve roots.[11,36] In the anterograde approach, the introducer needle is directed through either the interlaminar space or the sacral hiatus using a loss-of-resistance technique. This also can be done through a small laminectomy if percutaneous attempts are unsuccessful. Once the epidural space is entered, the electrode is passed rostrally and then directed laterally over the desired dorsal rootlets.[11,32,38]

Transforaminal nerve root stimulation is accomplished by means of the retrograde percutaneous approach. In this approach, the introducer needle is directed into the epidural space and the electrode passed in a caudal direction and steered into the appropriate neural foramen.[11,32,37] Typically, most patients who have pelvic pain syndromes respond most favorably to bilateral S-2 or S-3 electrodes. Placement in the L3 and L4 foramina results in stimulation

paresthesias focused along the knee, whereas L5 and S1 placement targets the foot. Thus, painful nerve injuries in these locations that prove refractory to less invasive measures may be treated effectively with transforaminal nerve root stimulation.

The trans-spinal technique[11,37,39] involves placement of an electrode into the neural foramen from a contralateral approach. In this technique, the introducer needle is placed in a paramedian fashion on the side contralateral to the desired neural foramen to be accessed. This may be done through either a percutaneous or open approach. The needle is advanced through the interlaminar space oriented parallel to the direction of the targeted nerve root. The epidural space is accessed at the midline, and the electrode then is advanced out laterally through the neural foramen and adjacent to the nerve root (**Fig. 7**). Because the cervical and thoracic nerve roots exit the spinal canal in a rather perpendicular fashion relative to the spinal cord, unlike the lumbosacral nerve roots, which are oriented more parallel, the trans-spinal technique theoretically offers anatomic advantages in accessing the nerve roots in these regions, which has proved difficult using the more traditional transforaminal or intraspinal techniques.

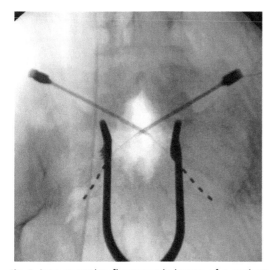

Fig. 7. Intraoperative fluoroscopic image of a patient during placement of bilateral trans-spinal nerve root electrodes at the S1 level used to treat tibial neuralgia. The S1 nerve roots were chosen, because the patient's pain was concentrated along the bottoms of the feet. An earlier trial of spinal cord stimulation was unsuccessful. The epidural space was accessed through a small midline laminectomy. Each electrode was placed through a small stab incision on the contralateral side, aiming in the direction of the target nerve root foramen. Note placement of the electrodes within the neural foramen, in a position overlying both the spinal nerve root and the dorsal root ganglion. As for each of these neurostimulation techniques, this may be done through either a percutaneous or an open approach.

Limitations

The limitations and contraindications to SNRS generally depend on the technique used for placement, although for all of the techniques there is a modestly added risk (beyond the standard risks of traditional SCS placement) of injury to the nerve root itself.[32] Although there may be particular advantages to the use of the trans-spinal technique in the cervicothoracic spine as previously discussed, access to the upper cervical spine above C-5 is contraindicated because of the risk of vertebral artery injury.[37] The most notable limitation for all of these SNRS techniques is a comparative lack of published outcome data for their use. The authors advocate their use by experienced practitioners in neurostimulation methods for specific applications not effectively addressed by more conventional forms of stimulation. A classic example is the use of SCS to treat upper extremity pain, and the supplemental use of a C6-8 intraspinal nerve root stimulator to provide augmented coverage of the hand that may remain uncovered by SCS alone.

SUBCUTANEOUS PERIPHERAL NERVE STIMULATION
Description

Occasionally, patients have pain that cannot be covered adequately by SCS, PNS, or SNRS techniques. In these cases, initial success has been reported using stimulator leads placed subcutaneously in the exact area or region of pain.[40–45] Often this technique is used in conjunction with an implanted SCS or PNS to provide adjunctive coverage of a focal area of pain.

Indications

Clinical reports of SPNS in the limb, inguinal area, and abdomen demonstrate its utility as a primary therapeutic modality.[40–42] In one report, Paicius and colleagues[40] demonstrated significant improvement in quality of life and reduction in opioid requirements following SPNS in patients who had inguinal neuralgia, chronic pancreatitis, and abdominal pain following liver transplantation, all of whom had failed nerve blocks, neurolysis, and medical therapy. In another small series, Goroszeniuk and colleagues[41] reported success in treating patients who had anterior chest wall and intercostal pain following various thoracic surgical procedures. They found that SPNS of 1 to 2 hours daily produced pain relief lasting 12 to 24 hours. Interestingly, these effects of SPNS did not correlate with transcutaneous electrical nerve stimulation, which none of the patients reported to be of any benefit. The authors have used SPNS in the treatment of postamputation stump pain when SCS failed to achieve the appropriate coverage along the painful area (**Fig. 8**).

In the case of chronic abdominal pain, SPNS may be uniquely advantageous, because this pain is often both neuropathic and nociceptive, and peripheral field stimulation covers both the regional dermatomal and visceral innervations that converge at the same spinal cord segment or segments, without the risk of neurologic sequelae possible with SCS. In fact, when SPNS is considered versus SCS in any situation, it offers the significant advantage of avoiding the spinal cord and associated risk of dural compromise and cord or root injury.[40,42] Preliminary studies have suggested that SPNS is quite useful as an adjunct treatment in concert with SCS.[46] For example, in patients who have FBSS and persistent low back and leg pain, SCS often effectively treats the lower extremity component of pain, but provides suboptimal relief for the low back pain. In these cases, the addition of subcutaneous electrodes may provide the necessary stimulation paresthesias and subsequent pain relief in the low back area (**Fig. 9**).

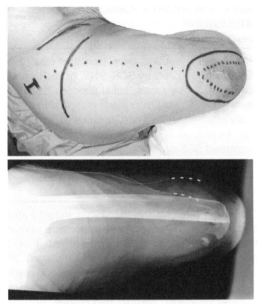

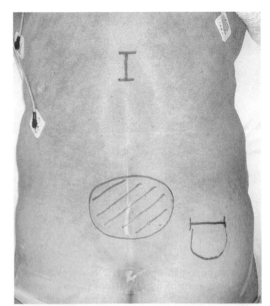

Fig. 8. Intraoperative radiograph (*above*) and postoperative radiograph (*below*) of a patient who underwent placement of subcutaneous peripheral nerve electrodes used to treat postamputation stump pain, located within the encircled region at the distal portion of the limb, adjacent to his healed incision. The curved line along the proximal hip represents the proximal extent of his prosthesis. The authors externalized his trial electrodes proximal to this point so that the prosthesis would not irritate the wires as they exited his skin. This patient had failed an earlier trial of spinal cord stimulation.

Technique

In SPNS, leads are placed subcutaneously at the specific area of pain, with local anesthesia. A trial of stimulation is performed similar to other forms of stimulation. If results are satisfactory, the temporary leads are discarded; permanent leads are placed and then connected to an implantable pulse generator. Most commonly, buttock or subcostal sites are chosen for the implantable pulse generator, depending upon location of the electrodes and patient preference. In cases where an existing PNS or SCS has been implanted and providing desirable coverage in all but a focal area of pain, and an SPNS is being used to cover that specific area, the lead is tunneled to the existing pulse generator.

Limitations

The primary limitation of SPNS is the lack of randomized–control studies or large case series demonstrating its efficacy and potential advantage to existing neuromodulation techniques. Although the preliminary results are promising, larger trials

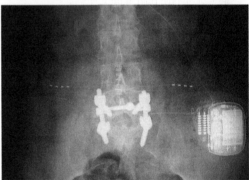

Fig. 9. Intraoperative radiograph (*above*) and postoperative radiograph (*below*) of a patient with failed back surgery syndrome and persistent low back and leg pain. During the spinal cord stimulator trial, the patient obtained excellent relief of the leg pain, but insufficient relief of the low back pain. The authors therefore placed a permanent low-thoracic spinal cord stimulator array (out of the field of view) to get leg coverage and added a supplemental array of subcutaneous peripheral nerve stimulator electrodes along the area of low back pain (*cross-hatched area on the skin*).

are necessary to establish this technique firmly among the neurostimulation options available to the surgeon today. Meanwhile, this may represent an excellent treatment option because of its ease of placement, few risks, and compatibility with existing stimulator systems.

REFERENCES

1. Mitchell SW, Morehouse CR, Keen WW. Gunshot wounds and other injuries of the nerves. Philadelphia: JB Lippincott; 1864. p. 143–57.

2. Melzack R, Wall PD. Pain mechanisms: a new theory. Science 1965;150(699):971–9.
3. Wall PD, Sweet WH. Temporary abolition of pain in man. Science 1967;155:108–9.
4. Shealy CN, Mortimer JT, Reswick J. Electrical inhibition of pain by stimulation of the dorsal column: preliminary clinical reports. Anesth Analg 1967;46: 489–91.
5. Lee AW, Pilitsis JG. Spinal cord stimulation: indications and outcomes. Neurosurg Focus 2006; 21(6):E3, 1–6.
6. Burchiel KJ, Anderson VC, Brown FD, et al. Prospective, multicenter study of spinal cord stimulation for relief of chronic back and extremity pain. Spine 1996;21:2786–94.
7. Kemler MA, Barendse GA, van Kleef M, et al. Spinal cord stimulation in patients with chronic reflex sympathetic dystrophy. N Engl J Med 2000;343:618–24.
8. North RB, Kidd DH, Farrokhi F, et al. Spinal cord stimulation versus repeated lumbosacral spine surgery for chronic pain: a randomized, controlled trial. Neurosurgery 2005;56:98–106.
9. North R, Shipley J, Prager J, et al. American Academy of Pain Medicine. Practice parameters for the use of spinal cord stimulation in the treatment of chronic neuropathic pain. Pain Med 2007;8(Suppl 4): S200–75.
10. Alo KM, Holsheimer J. New trends in neuromodulation for the management of neuropathic pain. Neurosurgery 2002;50:690–704.
11. Haque R, Winfree CJ. Spinal nerve root stimulation. Neurosurg Focus 2006;21(6):E4, 1–7.
12. Khan YN, Raza SS, Khan AE. Application of spinal cord stimulation for the treatment of abdominal visceral pain syndromes: case reports. Neuromodulation 2005;8(1):14–27.
13. Dunteman E. Peripheral nerve stimulation for unremitting ophthalmic postherpetic neuralgia. Neuromodulation 2002;5:32–7.
14. Johnson MD, Burchiel KJ. Peripheral stimulation for treatment of trigeminal postherpetic neuralgia and trigeminal post-traumatic neuropathic pain: a pilot study. Neurosurgery 2004;55:135–42.
15. Slavin KV, Burchiel KJ. Peripheral nerve stimulation for painful nerve injuries. Contemp Neurosurg 1999;21(19):1–6.
16. Slavin KV, Burchiel KJ. Use of long-term nerve stimulation with implanted electrodes in the treatment of intractable craniofacial pain. J Neurosurg 2000;92: 576 [abstract #827].
17. Slavin KV, Nersesyan H, Wess C. Treatment of neuropathic craniofacial pain using peripheral nerve stimulation approach. In: Meglio M, Krames ES, editors. Proceedings of 7th Meeting of International Neuromodulation Society, Rome (Italy), June 10–13, 2005. Bologna (Italy): Medimond; 2005. p. 77–80.
18. Slavin KV, Wess C. Trigeminal branch stimulation for intractable neuropathic pain: technical note. Neuromodulation 2005;8:7–13.
19. Nörenberg E, Winkelmuller W. The epifacial electric stimulation of the occipital nerve in cases of therapy-resistant neuralgia of the occipital nerve. Schmerz 2001;15:197–9 [German].
20. Hammer M, Doleys DM. Perineuromal stimulation in the treatment of occipital neuralgia: a case study. Neuromodulation 2001;4:47–52.
21. Kapural L, Mekhail N, Hayek SM, et al. Occipital nerve electrical stimulation via the midline approach and subcutaneous surgical leads for treatment of severe occipital neuralgia: a pilot study. Anesth Analg 2005;101:171–4.
22. Lou L. Uncommon areas of electrical stimulation. Curr Rev Pain 2000;4:407–12.
23. Slavin KV, Colpan ME, Munawar N, et al. Trigeminal and occipital peripheral nerve stimulation for craniofacial pain: a single-institution experience and review of the literature. Neurosurg Focus 2006; 21(6):E6, 1–5.
24. Slavin KV, Nersesyan H, Wess C. Peripheral neurostimulation for treatment of intractable occipital neuralgia. Neurosurgery 2006;58:112–9.
25. Magis D, Allena M, Bolla M, et al. Occipital nerve stimulation for drug-resistant chronic cluster headache: a prospective pilot study. Lancet Neurol 2007;6:314–21.
26. Weiner RL. Occipital neurostimulation for treatment of intractable headache syndromes. Acta Neurochir Suppl 2007;97:129–33.
27. Weiner RL. Peripheral nerve neurostimulation. Neurosurg Clin N Am 2003;14:401–8.
28. Rodrigo-Royo MD, Azcona JM, Quero J, et al. Peripheral neurostimulation in the management of cervicogenic headaches: four case reports. Neuromodulation 2005;8:241–8.
29. Alo KM, Gohel R, Corey CL. Sacral nerve root stimulation for the treatment of urge incontinence and detrusor dysfunction utilizing a cephalocaudal intraspinal method of lead insertion: a case report. Neuromodulation 2001;4:53–8.
30. Feler CA, Whitworth LA, Fernandez J. Sacral neuromodulation for chronic pain conditions. Anesthesiol Clin North America 2003;21:785–95.
31. Comiter CV. Sacral neuromodulation for the symptomatic treatment of refractory interstitial cystitis: a prospective study. J Urol 2003;169:1369–73.
32. Maher CF, Carey MP, Dwyer PL, et al. Percutaneous sacral nerve root neuromodulation for intractable interstitial cystitis. J Urol 2001;165:884–6.
33. Whitmore KE, Payne CK, Diokno AC, et al. Sacral neuromodulation in patients with interstitial cystitis: a multicenter clinical trial. Int Urogynecol J Pelvic Floor Dysfunct 2003;14:305–9.

34. Yearwood TL. Intraspinal nerve root stimulation for the treatment of axial lumbar spine pain in postlaminotomy syndrome. Presented at the 7th Meeting of the International Neuromodulation Society. Rome, Italy, June 10–13, 2005.

35. Yearwood TL. Neuropathic extremity pain and spinal cord stimulation. Pain Med 2006;7(Suppl 1): S97–102.

36. Alo KM, Yland MJ, Feler C, et al. A study of electrode placement at the cervical and upper thoracic nerve roots using an anatomic trans-spinal approach. Neuromodulation 1999;2:222–7.

37. Alo KM, Yland MJ, Redko V, et al. Lumbar and sacral nerve root stimulation (NRS) in the treatment of chronic pain: a novel anatomic approach and neurostimulation technique. Neuromodulation 1999;2: 23–31.

38. Falco FJ, Rubbani M, Heinbaugh J. Anterograde sacral nerve root stimulation (AS-NRS) via the sacral hiatus: benefits, limitations, and percutaneous implantation technique. Neuromodulation 2003;6: 219–24.

39. Urban BJ, Nashold BS Jr. Combined epidural and peripheral nerve stimulation for relief of pain. Description of technique and preliminary results. J Neurosurg 1982;57:365–9.

40. Pacius PM, Bernstein CA, Lempert-Cohen C. Peripheral nerve field stimulation in chronic abdominal pain. Pain Physician 2006;9:261–6.

41. Goroszeniuk T, Kothari S, Hamann W. Subcutaneous neuromodulating implant targeted at the site of pain. Reg Anesth Pain Med 2006;31:168–71.

42. Goroszeniuk T. Percutaneous insertion of permanent peripheral stimulating electrode in patients with neuropathic pain. Presented at the 6th World Congress of International Neuromodulation Society. Madrid, Spain, June 25–28, 2003.

43. Goroszeniuk T, Kothari S. Targeted external area stimulation. Reg Anesth Pain Med 2004;29(Suppl 2): 98–103.

44. Monti E. Peripheral nerve stimulation: a percutaneous minimally invasive approach. Neuromodulation 2004;7(3):193–6.

45. Stinson LW, Roderer GT, Cross NE, et al. Peripheral subcutaneous electrostimulation for control of intractible postoperative inguinal pain: a case report series. Neuromodulation 2001;4(3):99–104.

46. Bernstein CA, Paicius RM, Barkow SH, et al. Spinal cord stimulation in conjunction with peripheral nerve field stimulation for the treatment of low back and leg pain: a case series. Neuromodulation 2008;11: 116–23.

Peripheral Nerve: What's New in Basic Science Laboratories

Jae W. Song, MD[a], Lynda J. Yang, MD, PhD[b],
Stephen M. Russell, MD[a],*

KEYWORDS

- Nerve regeneration • Allotransplantation
- Electrical stimulation • Preferential motor reinneravation
- Transgenic mice

Peripheral nerve regeneration research reflects the historical events that have evolved understanding of this complex phenomenon. Over time, the works of clinicians and scientists have contributed insights into ways of optimizing repair. Two such examples are Sunderland and Rays'[1,2] seminal work in intraneural anatomy, which provided a map for the surgeon performing intrafascicular nerve repair, and on a cellular level, Cajal's contribution to neurohistology, much of which has been repeated, verified, and expanded upon by more sophisticated molecular and cellular biology techniques. Hence, research today aims to combine clinical expertise with the basic sciences. The group of investigators assembled during the Second World War by the Medical Research Council exemplifies the success of multidisciplinary investigations. Headed by Hugh Cairns and Herbert Seddon, professors of surgery at Oxford University, the team was joined by J.Z. Young,[3] a neuroscientist, who then recruited Ernst Gutmann, a Czech physician, Ludwig Guttmann, a neurologist, and Peter B. Medawar, a scientist who subsequently went on to win the Nobel Prize for his work on transplant research. Together, this multidisciplinary group, along with others, went on to make significant contributions in understanding function and pathology of peripheral nerves, highlighting the importance of translational basic science research.

In this article, the authors have chosen to discuss some current translational research in peripheral nerve regeneration. The article summarizes the research of nerve allotransplantation, which is founded upon principles of immunology and transplant biology.[4–6] It also discusses brief electrical stimulation after nerve repair as a new clinical therapy aimed to increase the rate of axonal regeneration. Lastly, it discusses current tools generated by neuroscientists that enable physicians to observe dynamic neurobiological processes at the cellular level, which may enable practitioners to answer clinical questions that were not answerable before.

PERIPHERAL NERVE ALLOTRANSPLANTATION

Nerve repair techniques in the early 19th century reflected the lack of biological understanding of nerve regeneration. Nerves, treated like elastic rubber bands, either were stretched[7] or patients' limbs specifically positioned[8] or shortened to approximate two nerve stumps. Later, secondary explorations of stretched nerves[9] and the lack of functional recovery suggested that better methodology was necessary. Philipeaux and Vulpian[10,11] are known to be the first to try both nerve allograft and nerve autografts in dogs. They described failure in allograft but some success with nerve autograft. In subsequent decades and with the

[a] Department of Neurosurgery, New York University School of Medicine, 462 First Avenue NB 7S-4, New York, NY 10016, USA
[b] Department of Neurosurgery, University of Michigan School of Medicine, 3552 Taubman Center, 1500 East Medical Center Drive, Ann Arbor, MI 48109, USA
* Corresponding author.
E-mail address: russes01@yahoo.com (S.M. Russell).

Neurosurg Clin N Am 20 (2009) 121–131
doi:10.1016/j.nec.2008.07.026
1042-3680/08/$ – see front matter © 2008 Elsevier Inc. All rights reserved.

casualties of World War I, autografts, xenografts, and allografts were re-evaluated extensively, and in the late 1940s, autogenous nerve grafts were established as the gold standard for nerve repair.[12] This procedure necessitates donor site morbidity, however, and hence other modalities have been explored, one of which is allografts. Peripheral nerve allotransplantation solves the problem of creating another intentional site of morbidity and provides, in theory, a limitless supply of nerve graft material. The first human nerve allotransplantation was performed by Albert in 1885[13] to reconstruct a large median and ulnar nerve gap from an amputated foot and leg. This unsuccessful attempt[14] was followed by many more disappointing results,[15] largely because of the lack of knowledge on transplantation immunology.

In the 1940s, Medawar and colleagues'[16] work on immunologic tolerance laid the groundwork for understanding the mechanism behind graft rejection, and with the advent of microneurosurgical techniques,[17] an interest in nerve allotransplantation was revived. First, various nerve allograft pretreatment and preservation methods were investigated. In the 1960s, systemic immunosuppression was introduced with the first clinical success of azathioprine for renal transplantation. Exploring combinations of different therapeutic modalities (ie, pretreatment and systemic immunosuppression) demonstrated synergistic advantages. Donor-specific tolerance (inducing tolerance specifically to allograft antigens in an otherwise immunocompetent patient) is a very attractive therapeutic modality that is being investigated.

Pretreatment and Storage

Storage methods were of interest, particularly during periods of war, because the possibility to preserve allograft material would provide the surgeon with ample material to treat war casualties in the time of need. With better understanding of the immune response, pretreatment methods aimed to preserve the graft for a length of time and reduce immunogenicity. Pretreatment methods that have been investigated include:

> Irradiation[18,19]
> Cryopreservation (deep-freezing)[20]
> Lyophilization (freeze-drying)[21,22]
> Freeze–thawing (repeated cycles of freezing [-70°C] and thawing [37°C] to render the graft acellular, leaving behind only the Schwann's cell basal lamina as a scaffold)[23]
> Predegeneration (allow donor nerve to degenerate in situ and allow time for Wallerian

degeneration to optimize neurotropic factors before harvest)[24,25]

Most of these pretreatment methods reduced antigenicity; however, nerve regeneration remained inferior compared with autografts.[26] Acellularizing the graft was one of the problems. Sustaining viable Schwann's cells until the graft is repopulated with host Schwann's cells is a critical feature in promoting nerve regeneration across the graft. Although short nerve gaps (less than 3 cm) can be bridged by acellular grafts,[27,28] longer defects are dependent on Schwann's cells and the molecular factors they release, which promote nerve regeneration. Cold preservation (at 2°C in Ringer's solution) of nerve allografts was investigated as a means of storage nearly 50 years ago[8,29] and was observed to sustain some viable Schwann's cells while reducing lymphocytic reaction. More recently, Mackinnon and colleagues[30,31] have extensively investigated cold preservation[32] of nerve allografts in University of Wisconsin (UW) storage solution (supplemented with penicillin, insulin, and dexamethasone). Storage at 5°C for a prolonged period (up to 3 weeks) both minimized antigenicity and sustained some viable Schwann's cells in rats.[31] In vitro assays of human nerve grafts revealed that cold preservation in UW storage solution for 7 days was most optimal for sustaining viable Schwann's cells, with decreasing populations of viable cells with storage longer than 7 days.[31] These are promising results for delineating the conditions with which nerve allografts may be optimally pretreated. For longer peripheral nerve defects, however, it remains a problem to sustain graft Schwann's cells until both the regenerating axon and comigrating host Schwann's cells can repopulate the graft. Current investigations addressing this problem include seeding cultured autologous Schwann's cells within nerve allografts.[33] Preliminary studies report significant regeneration along 6 cm nerve defects in a primate model using this paradigm.

Host Immunosuppression

As opposed to pretreatment methods, an alternative strategy is suppressing the host's immunity, which would leave all components of the graft (cells and structural elements, ie, basal lamina) intact and viable. The success of systemic immunosuppression first was demonstrated in renal transplantation, and its success in the 1960s provided a turning point in transplantation surgery. Soon various immunosuppressant therapies were investigated. Borel and colleagues[34] first introduced cyclosporin A to the field as an immunosuppressant in 1976. Cyclosporin A prevents interleukin (IL)-2 synthesis, a potent T-cell activator and proliferating cytokine, thus generating a nonspecific immunosuppressed state with less lymphotoxicity than most other immunosuppressant's.[35] It soon became the drug of choice for patients who had allografted organs,[36] and subsequently also was tested for nerve allograft experiments. A minimum effective dose and regimen to prevent graft rejection and its ability to allow regeneration through allografts were assayed in systemically immunosuppressed rodent models.[37–40] Histomorphometric, electrophysiologic, and sciatic nerve functional indices of nerve regeneration were assayed in rats grafted with 3 cm long allografts treated with and without daily doses (5 mg/kg/d) of cyclosporin A, and by 14 weeks after grafting, allografts were statistically indistinguishable from syngeneic (equivalent to receiving an autograft) controls.[39] These studies were repeated in primates,[41,42] and also in sheep using longer (8 cm) nerve allograft material.[43] Cyclosporin A successfully demonstrated histologic evidence of axon regeneration in allografts.

Recipients of organ transplants typically receive life-long systemic immunosuppressant therapy. Unlike transplanted visceral organs, however, peripheral nerve allografts are unique. Ideally, the transplanted allograft only is masked for a temporary period with immunosuppression therapy while providing a scaffold and milieu for host axons and cells to repopulate the graft. With this in mind, short-term immunosuppression was investigated, and in fact, found to be sufficient for axons to regenerate and prevent graft rejection.[44–46] Although cyclosporin A appeared effective for preventing graft rejection, it did not enhance nerve regeneration. For long defects, the ideal agent would promote nerve regeneration and have immunosuppressive properties. Thus, other immunosuppressive agents were investigated. One such drug investigated was FK506 (tacrolimus).

FK506, similar to cyclosporin A, inhibits synthesis of IL-2, resulting in systemic nonspecific immunosuppression. FK506 was first tested by Buttemeyer and colleagues[47,48] and reported as a possible alternative to cyclosporin A. It was discovered that FK506 was significantly more effective in stimulating nerve regeneration while concurrently preventing graft rejection.[49] This study was repeated in a swine model with a longer nerve allograft (8 cm), and similar results were found,[50] verifying FK506 as an immunosuppressant and regeneration-enhancing agent. Studies suggest that FK506 stimulates neural regeneration by increasing GAP-43 mRNA,[51] promoting collateral sprouting,[52] and acting as a neurotrophic agent.[53] Studies are being conducted to investigate whether subimmunosuppressive doses of FK506 can enhance axon regeneration rates or nonimmunosuppressive analogs of FK506 would be effective in enhancing axon regeneration.

Combination therapies also have been explored. The most effective combination therapy was apparent with the combination of cold preservation in UW storage solution and systemic immunosuppression using FK506 in a murine model. Doses of FK506 were reduced, and axonal regeneration was observed to be statistically indistinguishable from autografts. Moreover, regeneration exceeded regeneration in nerve autografts, revealing it as a regeneration-enhancing agent.[54]

Clinical Trials

MacKinnon and colleagues[44,55,56] have applied decades of research on nerve allotransplantation to the clinical setting. In their first case report, an 8-year-old boy received 10 cable nerve grafts (23 cm in length) to his left sciatic nerve.[44] He received oral cyclosporin A and oral prednisone for 26 months after surgery, until functional sensibility in the peroneal and posterior tibial nerve distribution was observed. In this case, some sensory recovery was obtained, but no motor recovery was observed. This was attributed to the lengthy defect the motor axons needed to cross to reach the target muscle, which progressively became denervated. In a subsequent clinical study, seven patients (mean age, 15 years; range 3 to 24 years) were managed with allografts or a combination of autografts and allografts by cable grafting techniques.[56] Allografts were matched for donor and recipient blood types, harvested, and preserved in UW storage solution at 5°C for 7 days to minimize antigenicity. Patients were immunosuppressed with either a combination of prednisone, azathioprine, and cyclosporin A (n = 5) or in place of cyclosporin A, FK506 (n = 2) for an average of 18.5 months (range 12 to 26 months). In one patient, rejection of an allograft occurred because of subtherapeutic levels of cyclosporin A. All other patients, however, demonstrated some sensory and/or motor recovery.

PROMOTING REGENERATION WITH ELECTRICAL STIMULATION

All endeavors to enhance peripheral nerve regeneration must deal with the critical issue of time and distance. Regardless of therapeutic modality used to repair an injured nerve, the proximal end of the nerve stump regenerates at a relatively slow rate. This delay is problematic, with recent studies demonstrating an optimal regenerative (axon) and receptive (target end organ) time window, after which both components progressively lose their capacity to fully recover function.

The effects on functional recovery of prolonged motor neuron axotomy and prolonged muscle denervation were evaluated independently after delayed (up to one year) nerve repair.[57,58] These authors used nerve cross-anastomosis in the rabbit hind limb, an experimental procedure first introduced by Holmes and Young (1942). In brief, to evaluate the ability of chronically axotomized regenerating motor neurons to reinnervate freshly denervated muscle, they first transected the posterior tibial nerve and sutured it to the innervated lateral gastrocnemius muscle, to preclude regeneration. A second surgery was performed after varying time intervals (up to 1 year), where the previously ligated tibial nerve was cross-sutured to the distal end of a cut common peroneal nerve, innervating the tibialis anterior muscle. Alternatively, to evaluate the effect of chronic muscle denervation, the common peroneal nerve was transected, and regeneration was prevented by suturing it to the biceps femoris. The tibialis anterior muscle was left denervated for up to 1 year before the tibial nerve was cut and a tibial-common peroneal cross-anastomosis was performed. Nerve regeneration and muscle reinnervation were evaluated using electrophysiologic and histologic methods to quantify muscle and motor unit forces. Chronically denervated muscles (ie, longer than 6 months) became progressively less receptive to regenerating axons. Theoretically, the lack of neurotrophic factors after a prolonged delay may prevent maintenance of functional contacts or synapses. This translated into a 90% reduction of the number of functional motor units after 6 months of denervation. In addition to the deleterious effects of chronic muscle denervation, the Schwann's cells from the distal nerve branch also progressively become chronically denervated.[59] Typically after nerve injury, the distal Schwann's cells clear the distal pathways of degenerating axon and myelin debris by phagocytosis and digestion. These cells then proliferate in alignment using a configuration known as "Bands of Bunger" and await regenerating axons. During this regenerative interim, these Schwann's cells up-regulate a molecular array of growth-associated proteins that promote axon growth.[60] Unfortunately, this period of receptiveness is limited. In vivo studies in rodents reveal that chronically denervated Schwann's cells eventually atrophy and become progressively refractory to the milieu of regenerating axons.[60] After prolonged axotomy, (especially beyond 3 months) a significantly reduced number of motor axons

regenerated.[58] The axons that did regenerate, however, tended to reinnervate muscle fibers by expanding their motor unit size. In summary, these studies revealed a limited time period after which functional recovery was limited severely. Thus, efforts should be dedicated to increasing the number of regenerating motor neurons or sustaining the receptiveness of the denervated muscle and Schwann's cells to improve regeneration and functional recovery. In reality, these two phenomena occur in parallel. Moreover, in people, the large distance that axons must traverse to reach the target end organs is prohibitive,[61] further emphasizing the critical issue of time.

Rate of Nerve Regeneration

Interest in the rate of nerve regeneration first was addressed histologically by Cajal[62] and independently described in the clinical setting in 1915 by Tinel[63,64] and Hoffman.[65] In the 1940s, a more complete and systematic study of the rate of nerve regeneration in rabbits[66] and people[67] was investigated. Regeneration is described as occurring in three steps:[67]

(1) An initial delay at the suture or scar site (comprising the latent or lag period).
(2) Mature axons traversing the distance toward the end organ.
(3) The time required for the fibers to reestablish functionality at the muscle or skin.

Although it generally is accepted that nerves regenerate at a rate of 1 mm/d, recent studies have demonstrated a much more protracted period of regeneration.[68] In a rodent model, the femoral nerve was transected and repaired, and the muscle nerve branch was back-labeled with neurotracers after a period of 2 to 10 weeks to identify regenerating motor neurons. The neurotracers were applied 25 mm from the original repair site. If all nerves regenerated at 1 mm/d, by 4 weeks, most of the regenerating motor neurons should be back-labeled. Surprisingly, 8 to 10 weeks passed before most of the motor neurons traversed the length of the defect. This dramatic result was putatively attributed to characteristic collateral sprouting that occurs with regenerating axons.[69] These sprouts appear to emerge from nearby nodes of Ranvier.[70,71] As nutrient resources are distributed down each of these sprouts, the rate of regeneration may be slowed until these collaterals are pruned, and material is focused down the regenerating parent axon. Second, the suture site, where there is considerable scarring, appears to significantly contribute to this delay.[66,72,73] Axons regenerate asynchronously across this suture site, and a significant amount of wandering, both laterally and retrograde into the proximal nerve stump, occurs at the scarred region before axon collaterals enter a distal endoneurial tube.[62,74] Studies demonstrated a differential regenerative ability among motor neurons, with only 25% of motor axons traversing the suture site by 7 days. This largely asynchronous and variable ability of motor axons to regenerate has been described as staggered regeneration.[75–77]

In efforts to promote regeneration and compress this period of delay, the influence of electrical stimulation in promoting axon growth has been evaluated.[68,73,78] Results revealed that the delay in nerve regeneration could be reduced to 3 weeks after 1 hour of 20 Hz continuous electrical stimulation, in striking contrast to the 8 to 10 weeks required without electrical stimulation.[68] Using neurotracers to label regenerated axons that had just crossed the surgical repair site, a follow-up study demonstrated an accelerated recruitment of regenerating motor axons across the injury site when electrical stimulation was used. There was, however, no increase in the rate of slow axonal transport, which reflects the regeneration rate.[73] When tetrodotoxin was applied to prevent action potential transmissions, the effects of electrical stimulation on regeneration vanished, suggesting the mechanism was mediated in the cell body, perhaps by gene transcription regulation.[68] Using semiquantitative in situ hybridization, indeed a more rapid and robust mRNA expression of the neurotrophin, brain-derived neurotrophic factor (BDNF) and its high-affinity receptor trkB were observed in regenerating motor axons after 1 hour of 20 Hz electrical stimulation, in contrast to controls not receiving electrical stimulation.[79] Moreover, this transcriptional response was followed by an increase in mRNA expression levels of regeneration-associated genes (eg, alpha1-tubulin and GAP-43), which also were elevated significantly by electrical stimulation compared with controls. This result suggests that BDNF/trkB signaling regulates gene expression of cytoskeletal proteins, which acts to promote the outgrowth of growth cones in regenerating motor axons.[80]

Reinnervation Specificity

These studies also addressed another critical issue that frequently complicates complete recovery: the misdirection of regenerating motor and sensory nerves. This random reinnervation, which contributes to poor functional recovery has been documented both experimentally[81] and clinically.[82] Using the femoral nerve paradigm and a double-retrograde labeling technique, Brushart and Seiler[75,77] investigated the specificity with which motor axons regenerated toward their targets. Surprisingly, given equal access to motor and sensory pathways, regenerating motor axons appeared to selectively reinnervate motor pathways. During early stages of regeneration (3 to 4 weeks), motor axons sent an equal number of collaterals to both motor and sensory pathways. During the later stages of regeneration (8 to 10 weeks), however, most motor axons were observed to reinnervate motor pathways, with fewer in the sensory pathways. This pattern was termed preferential motor reinnervation. This specificity is attributed to a pruning mechanism.[77] Motor axons incorrectly innervating sensory pathways somehow are recognized and pruned, whereas motor axons correctly innervating motor pathways are maintained. This specificity was observed even without the presence of the target end organ, suggesting that cues from the regenerating axons and Schwann's cells may be more critical for the emergence of preferential motor reinnervation.[76] The authors suggested that Schwann's cells maintained specific identities associated with their previously innervating axon type and thus were able to promote or maintain the same type of regenerating axon selectively. This was supported further by observing a differential ability of sensory axon-sheathing Schwann's cells versus motor axon-sheathing Schwann's cells to express a carbohydrate epitope (L2/HNK-1 carbohydrate; labeled by anti-L2 and anti-HNK-1 antibodies) when approached by regenerating motor axons. L2/HNK-1 carbohydrate rarely is expressed on Schwann's cells sheathing intact sensory axons, and when incorrectly reinnervated by motor axons, these Schwann's cells previously sheathing sensory axons only weakly express L2 carbohydrate. In contrast, robust L2/HNK-1 carbohydrate expression is seen on Schwann's cells previously innervating motor axons.[83] L2/HNK-1 carbohydrate acting as a possible motor axon specific recognition molecule or having a positive effect on regeneration is consistent with other studies. Schwann's cell-derived L2 promotes neurite outgrowth from motor neuron cultures[84] and is expressed selectively on Schwann's cells of motor axons but not sensory axons.[85] This may provide a mechanism by which regenerating motor axons may be maintained selectively in motor pathways. Moreover, brief electrical stimulation also appeared to improve the accuracy with which motor axons regenerated motor pathways. With brief electrical stimulation, the progressive increase in correctly reinnervating motor pathways was apparent by 3 weeks versus 8 weeks without electrical stimulation.[68] Electrical stimulation also increased L2/HNK-1 expression in the motor branch but appeared to have no such effect in the regenerating cutaneous branch.[86] This finding correlates with earlier and increased expression of BDNF and TrkB induced by electrical stimulation, suggesting BDNF/TrkB signaling modulates L2/HNK-1 expression in Schwann's cells, influencing preferential motor reinnervation.[86]

These studies demonstrate a potential clinical role for brief electrical stimulation in nerve repair. It appears to promote nerve regeneration across the surgical suture site and thus to decrease the time required for axons to traverse the length of the defect. Clearly, this is an advantage, as axons would reach the distal Schwann's cell tubes and muscles faster, lessening the effect of chronic denervation.[57,58] Gordon and colleagues[87,88] recently translated these findings from rat models to the clinical setting in a randomized–controlled trial of 21 people diagnosed with moderate-to-severe carpal tunnel syndrome who underwent operative carpal tunnel release. The number of reinnervated motor units in the median nerve-innervated thenar muscle before and after carpal tunnel release surgery was measured at varying intervals over the course of 12 months in subjects who had received low-frequency electrical stimulation for 1 hour immediately after the operation. Patients who received electrical stimulation after the surgery demonstrated a significant increase in motor axon regeneration in contrast to control patient groups, measured by the motor unit number estimates (MUNE). Associated with this result was an improvement in manual dexterity (Purdue Pegboard Test), reduced symptom severity (Levine Carpal Tunnel Syndrome Questionnaire), and improved sensation (Semmes-Weinstein Monofilaments).[87] These initial studies demonstrate the feasibility of clinically applying postsurgical electrical stimulation in people to accelerate and thus improve axon regeneration and functional outcomes in a crush injury.

ADVANCES IN NEUROSCIENCE RELEVANT TO PERIPHERAL NERVE

In vivo imaging of the nervous system recently began a new and exciting direction of study, which now enables practitioners to directly observe dynamic behavior of individual cells of the nervous system with higher temporal and spatial resolution. The coadvancement of optical microscopy and sophisticated mouse genetics now allows practitioners to directly observe the nervous system at the level of single cells in their native

milieu.[89–92] The recent generation of sophisticated transgenic mouse lines (Thy-1-XFP mice), which selectively express spectral variants of green fluorescent protein in neurons, have provided a new tool to study the nervous system. In these mice, neurons selectively express fluorescent proteins by direct control of a modified Thy-1 promoter.[91] In some of the Thy-1-XFP lines, because of the positional effects of gene insertion, the transgene expression is restricted to a smaller percentage of neurons, which is advantageous for some studies, in particular the densely innervated central nervous system. These lines are called subset lines (ie, Thy-1-YFP-H, Thy-1-CFP-S).[93] These transgenic mice enable practitioners to visualize and reconstruct axons in their entirety,[94] accurately identify the same axon over time,[95,96] and directly observe their dynamism in their native milieu.[97] Furthermore, by crossing mice expressing different colors of fluorescent proteins in a subset of their neurons, interactions between the two different cells are subject to analysis.[96] Previously, with single-color labeling techniques, such analysis was impossible. The discovery of the ability to genetically alter mice to visualize a specific cell type led to the generation of many other transgenic lines, which now include:

> Schwann's cells under the S100-promoter[98]
> Oligodendrocytes under the PLP-promoter[99]
> Macrophages and microglial cells by knocking in green fluorescent protein for the chemokine receptor CX_3CR1[100]
> Mitochondria (exclusively in neurons) under the Thy-1-coxVIII (mitochondrial targeting sequence from human cytochrome oxidase subunit VIII) promoter[91,101]

The ability to directly visualize these specific cell types that comprise the nervous system are an invaluable tool for providing insight into the diseased nervous system (eg, axonal regeneration and degeneration).

One of the primary advantages of using these mice is the ability to observe dynamism among the same cells in their native environment over time. A sequence of events in a cellular process can be observed directly rather than extrapolated from single time points using different animals. One study that exemplifies these advantages examined the fidelity with which axons after traumatic crush injury reinnervated the same target muscle fibers.[102] The advantages of using Thy-1 mice for this particular study are manifold. First, because of the bright fluorescence expressed by the axon, an injury inflicted upon the axon is confirmed directly by the lack of fluorescence with relative ease.[103] Second, the axon of interest is identified quickly and easily at each time point over a period of several days to a month to observe the reinnervation events. This study revealed that after a crush injury, axons reinnervated the same muscle fibers with remarkable precision, and the regenerating axons even branched at the same original branching points. Presumably the endoneurial tubes were intact after such a crush injury. In contrast, after complete transection of the axon (both axons and endoneurial tubes are discontinuous), not only was reinnervation of the muscle fibers incomplete, but regenerating axons were misrouted, often reinnervating synapses that were reinnervated previously by other motor axons. These observations emphasize that in addition to molecular cues, mechanical confinements play a role in directional specificity during regeneration of peripheral motor axons.[102]

Direct imaging of peripheral axons in real time after axotomy has provided more accurate assays of studying degenerating and regenerating nerves.[101] For instance, one now can measure axonal transport rates. Recent advances in visualizing neuronal mitochondrial dynamics in living mice (and hence measure organelle transport in axons) in real time has been accomplished with the generation of new lines of transgenic mice that express fluorescent protein exclusively in axonal mitochondria.[101] The unique polarity of neurons requires these highly specialized cells to have mechanisms that tightly regulate the allocation of nutrients and organelles to axonal branches situated far away from the cell body. Misgeld and colleagues[101] examined changes in axonal transport that accompany axon regeneration in acutely explanted peripheral nerve–muscle preparations. A robust increase in anterograde transport of mitochondria to the proximal end of the transected axon was observed even before visual evidence of axon regeneration. As growth cones advanced, mitochondria rapidly repopulated the distal-most region of the growth cone. This sudden increase in the anterograde transport rate was maintained for 48 hours and only declined minimally in the ensuing weeks. These results suggest the possibility of detecting axonal pathology earlier with changes in transport rates and may reflect a cell body response.[104] Axotomized peripheral neurons undergo immediate changes that are visible at the somal level and collectively are called chromatolysis. It is possible that these changes also are reflected in mitochondria rate of transport. Mitochondria are trafficked to areas of the axon where metabolic demand is high, such as actively growing axons.[105–110] Noting the changes in the rate of transport of organelles is now possible with these transgenic mice and in vivo imaging techniques, which are sensitive enough to acquire images in real-time.

SUMMARY

Currently, there is an emphasis in translating the knowledge of neurobiology obtained in the laboratory into practical clinical applications. The successful transition and application of both nerve allotransplantation and brief electrical stimulation into the clinical arena are examples of how this ultimate goal can be achieved. The vast enrichment of knowledge in the fields of immunology, neurobiology, molecular biology, and imaging techniques over the years provides mechanistic understanding, which is ultimately fundamental for improving potential clinical therapies. New tools generated by basic investigations, such as the Thy-1-XFP transgenic lines, already have become invaluable tools for investigating clinical questions in the field of peripheral nerve regeneration. Other exciting avenues of peripheral nerve regeneration research not discussed in this article include neural stem cells, tissue engineering, neurotrophic factors and pharmacologic agents, and neuroprosthetics. A multidisciplinary approach to research will prove most successful in the evolution of clinical applications with the goal of improving functional outcomes after nerve repair.

REFERENCES

1. Sunderland S. The intraneural topography of the radial, median, and ulnar nerves. Brain 1945;68: 243–98.
2. Sunderland S, Ray LJ. The intraneural topography of the sciatic nerve and its popliteal divisions in man. Brain 1948;71:242–73.
3. Young JZ. Introduction. In: Dyck PJ, Thomas PK, editors. Peripheral neuropathy. 3rd edition. Philadelphia: W.B. Saunders; 1993. p. 2–5.
4. Jensen JN, Mackinnon SE. Composite tissue allotransplantation: a comprehensive review of the literature—part 1. J Reconstr Microsurg 2000;16:57–68.
5. Jensen JN, Mackinnon SE. Composite tissue allotransplantation: a comprehensive review of the literature—part II. J Reconstr Microsurg 2000;16:141–57.
6. Jensen JN, Mackinnon SE. Composite tissue allotransplantation: a comprehensive review of the literature—part III. J Reconstr Microsurg 2000;16:235–51.
7. Richardson MH. Operations on nerves. Boston Medical and Surgical Journal 1886;115:368.
8. Schuller M. Die Verwendung der Nervendehnung zur operativen Heilung von Ubstanzverlusten am Nerven. Wien Med Presse 1888;29:145–52.

9. Stookey B. The futility of bridging nerve defects by means of nerve flaps. Surg Gynecol Obstet 1919; 29:287–311.

10. Philipeaux JM, Vulpian A. Recherches experimentales sur la reunion bout a bout de nerfs de fonctions differentes. Jounral Physiologie de L'Homme et L'Animal 1863;6:474–516.

11. Philipeaux JM, Vulpian A. Note sur des essais de greffe d'un troncon du nerf lingual entre les deux bouts du nerf hypoglosse, apres excision d'un segment de ce dernier nerf. Arch Physiol Norm Pathol 1870;3:618–20.

12. Seddon HJ. The use of autogenous grafts for the repair of large gaps in peripheral nerves. Br J Surg 1947;35:151–67.

13. Albert E. Einige operationen am nerven. Wien Med Presse 1885;26:1285.

14. Huber GC. A study of the operative treatment for loss of nerve substance in peripheral nerves. J Morphol 1895;11:629–735.

15. Sanders FK. The repair of large gaps in the peripheral nerves. Brain 1942;65:281–337.

16. Billingham RE, Brent L, Medawar PB. Actively acquired tolerance of foreign cells. Nature 1953; 172:603–6.

17. Millesi H. Microsurgical nerve grafting. Int Surg 1980;65:503–8.

18. Marmor L, Foster JM, Carlson GJ, et al. Experimental irradiated nerve heterografts. J Neurosurg 1966; 24:656–66.

19. Easterling KJ, Trumble TE. The treatment of peripheral nerve injuries using irradiated allografts and temporary host immunosuppression (in a rat model). J Reconstr Microsurg 1990;6:301–7.

20. Zalewski AA, Gulati AK. Evaluation of histocompatibility as a factor in the repair of nerve with a frozen nerve allograft. J Neurosurg 1982;56:550–4.

21. Weiss P. Functional nerve regeneration through frozen-dried nerve grafts in cats and monkeys. Proc Soc Exp Biol Med 1943;54:277–9.

22. Weiss P, Taylor C. Repair of peripheral nerves by grafts of frozen-dried nerve. Proc Soc Exp Biol Med 1943;52:326–8.

23. Wang GY, Hirai K, Shimada H. The role of laminin, a component of Schwann's cell basal lamina, in rat sciatic nerve regeneration within antiserum-treated nerve grafts. Brain Res 1992;570:116–25.

24. Bentley FH, Hill M. Nerve grafting. Br J Surg 1936; 24:368–87.

25. Trumble TE. Peripheral nerve transplantation: the effects of predegenerated grafts and immunosuppression. J Neural Transplant Plast 1992;3: 39–49.

26. Mackinnon SE, Hudson AR, Falk RE, et al. Peripheral nerve allograft: an assessment of regeneration across pretreated nerve allografts. Neurosurgery 1984;15:690–3.

27. Strauch B, Ferder M, Lovelle-Allen S, et al. Determining the maximal length of a vein conduit used as an interposition graft for nerve regeneration. J Reconstr Microsurg 1996;12:521–7.

28. Sanders FK, Young JZ. The degeneration and reinnervation of grafted nerves. J Anat 1942;76: 143–66.

29. Gutmann E, Sanders FK. Recovery of fibre numbers and diameters in the regeneration of peripheral nerves. J Physiol 1943;101:489–518.

30. Evans PJ, Mackinnon SE, Best TJ, et al. Regeneration across preserved peripheral nerve grafts. Muscle Nerve 1995;18:1128–38.

31. Levi AD, Evans PJ, Mackinnon SE, et al. Cold storage of peripheral nerves: an in vitro assay of cell viability and function. Glia 1994;10:121–31.

32. Belzer FO, Southard JH. Principles of solid-organ preservation by cold storage. Transplantation 1988;45:673–6.

33. Hess JR, Brenner MJ, Fox IK, et al. Use of cold-preserved allografts seeded with autologous Schwann's cells in the treatment of a long-gap peripheral nerve injury. Plast Reconstr Surg 2007; 119:246–59.

34. Borel JF, Feurer C, Gubler HU, et al. Biological effects of cyclosporin A: a new antilymphocytic agent. Agents Actions 1976;6:468–75.

35. Ruhlmann A, Nordheim A. Effects of the immunosuppressive drugs CsA and FK506 on intracellular signaling and gene regulation. Immunobiology 1997;198:192–206.

36. Cohen DJ, Loertscher R, Rubin MF, et al. Cyclosporine: a new immunosuppressive agent for organ transplantation. Ann Intern Med 1984;101:667–82.

37. Zalewski AA, Gulati AK. Survival of nerve allografts in sensitized rats treated with cyclosporin A. J Neurosurg 1984;60:828–34.

38. Zalewski AA, Gulati AK. Failure of cyclosporin A to induce immunological unresponsiveness to nerve allografts. Exp Neurol 1984;83:659–63.

39. Bain JR, Mackinnon SE, Hudson AR, et al. The peripheral nerve allograft: an assessment of regeneration across nerve allografts in rats immunosuppressed with cyclosporin A. Plast Reconstr Surg 1988;82: 1052–66.

40. Bain JR, Mackinnon SE, Hudson AR, et al. The peripheral nerve allograft: a dose–response curve in the rat immunosuppressed with cyclosporin A. Plast Reconstr Surg 1988;82:447–57.

41. Bain JR, Mackinnon SE, Hudson AR, et al. The peripheral nerve allograft in the primate immunosuppressed with cyclosporin A: I. Histologic and electrophysiologic assessment. Plast Reconstr Surg 1992;90:1036–46.

42. Fish JS, Bain JR, McKee N, et al. The peripheral nerve allograft in the primate immunosuppressed with cyclosporin A: II. Functional evaluation of

reinnervated muscle. Plast Reconstr Surg 1992;90: 1047–52.

43. Matsuyama T, Midha R, Mackinnon SE, et al. Long nerve allografts in sheep with cyclosporin A immunosuppression. J Reconstr Microsurg 2000;16:219–25.

44. Mackinnon SE, Midha R, Bain J, et al. An assessment of regeneration across peripheral nerve allografts in rats receiving short courses of cyclosporin A immunosuppression. Neuroscience 1992;46:585–93.

45. Midha R, Mackinnon SE, Evans PJ, et al. Comparison of regeneration across nerve allografts with temporary or continuous cyclosporin A immunosuppression. J Neurosurg 1993;78:90–100.

46. Atchabahian A, Doolabh VB, Mackinnon SE, et al. Indefinite survival of peripheral nerve allografts after temporary cyclosporin A immunosuppression. Restor Neurol Neurosci 1998;13:129–39.

47. Buttemeyer R, Jones NF, Rao UN. Peripheral nerve allotransplant immunosuppressed with FK 506: preliminary results. Transplant Proc 1995;27: 1877–8.

48. Buttemeyer R, Rao U, Jones NF. Peripheral nerve allograft transplantation with FK506: functional, histological, and immunological results before and after discontinuation of immunosuppression. Ann Plast Surg 1995;35:396–401.

49. Myckatyn TM, Ellis RA, Grand AG, et al. The effects of rapamycin in murine peripheral nerve isografts and allografts. Plast Reconstr Surg 2002;109: 2405–17.

50. Jensen JN, Brenner MJ, Tung TH, et al. Effect of FK506 on peripheral nerve regeneration through long grafts in inbred swine. Ann Plast Surg 2005; 54:420–7.

51. Gold BG, Yew JY, Zeleny-Pooley M. The immunosuppressant FK506 increases GAP-43 mRNA levels in axotomized sensory neurons. Neurosci Lett 1998;241:25–8.

52. Udina E, Ceballos D, Gold BG, et al. FK506 enhances reinnervation by regeneration and by collateral sprouting of peripheral nerve fibers. Exp Neurol 2003;183:220–31.

53. Steiner JP, Connolly MA, Valentine HL, et al. Neurotrophic actions of nonimmunosuppressive analogues of immunosuppressive drugs FK506, rapamycin, and cyclosporin A. Nat Med 1997;3:421–8.

54. Grand AG, Myckatyn TM, Mackinnon SE, et al. Axonal regeneration after cold preservation of nerve allografts and immunosuppression with tacrolimus in mice. J Neurosurg 2002;96:924–32.

55. Mackinnon SE. Nerve allotransplantation following severe tibial nerve injury. Case report. J Neurosurg 1996;84:671–6.

56. Mackinnon SE, Doolabh VB, Novak CB, et al. Clinical outcome following nerve allograft transplantation. Plast Reconstr Surg 2001;107:1419–29.

57. Fu SY, Gordon T. Contributing factors to poor functional recovery after delayed nerve repair: prolonged denervation. J Neurosci 1995;15:3886–95.

58. Fu SY, Gordon T. Contributing factors to poor functional recovery after delayed nerve repair: prolonged axotomy. J Neurosci 1995;15:3876–85.

59. Sulaiman OA, Gordon T. Effects of short- and long-term Schwann's cell denervation on peripheral nerve regeneration, myelination, and size. Glia 2000;32:234–46.

60. Hall SM. The biology of chronically denervated Schwann's cells. Ann N Y Acad Sci 1999;883:215–33.

61. Hoke A. Mechanisms of disease: what factors limit the success of peripheral nerve regeneration in humans? Nat Clin Pract Neurol 2006;2:448–54.

62. Ramon Y, Cajal S. Degeneration and regeneration of the nervous system [reprinted] 1991 edition. Oxford (UK): Oxford University Press; 1928.

63. Tinel J. Le signe du fourmillementdans les lésions des nerfs périphériques. Presse Medicale 1915; 47:388.

64. Tinel J. Tingling signs with peripheral nerve injuries. 1915. J Hand Surg [Br] 2005;30:87–9.

65. Hoffmann P, Buck-Gramcko D, Lubahn JD. The Hoffmann-Tinel sign. 1915. J Hand Surg [Br] 1993;18:800–5.

66. Gutmann E, Guttmann L, Medawar PB, et al. The rate of regeneration of nerve. J Exp Biol 1942;19: 14–44.

67. Seddon HJ, Medawar PB, Smith H. Rate of regeneration of peripheral nerves in man. J Physiol 1943; 102:191–215.

68. Al-Majed AA, Neumann CM, Brushart TM, et al. Brief electrical stimulation promotes the speed and accuracy of motor axonal regeneration. J Neurosci 2000;20:2602–8.

69. Aitken JT, Sharman M, Young JZ. Maturation of regenerating nerve fibres with various peripheral connexions. J Anat 1947;81:1–22.

70. Morris JH, Hudson AR, Weddell G. A study of degeneration and regeneration in the divided rat sciatic nerve based on electron microscopy. IV. Changes in fascicular microtopography, perineurium, and endoneurial fibroblasts. Z Zellforsch Mikrosk Anat 1972;124:165–203.

71. MacKinnon SE, Dellon AL, O'Brien JP. Changes in nerve fiber numbers distal to a nerve repair in the rat sciatic nerve model. Muscle Nerve 1991;14: 1116–21.

72. Forman DS, Wood DK, DeSilva S. Rate of regeneration of sensory axons in transected rat sciatic nerve repaired with epineurial sutures. J Neurol Sci 1979;44:55–9.

73. Brushart TM, Hoffman PN, Royall RM, et al. Electrical stimulation promotes motoneuron regeneration without increasing its speed or conditioning the neuron. J Neurosci 2002;22:6631–8.

74. Witzel C, Rohde C, Brushart TM. Pathway sampling by regenerating peripheral axons. J Comp Neurol 2005;485:183–90.

75. Brushart TM, Seiler WA 4th. Selective reinnervation of distal motor stumps by peripheral motor axons. Exp Neurol 1987;97:289–300.

76. Brushart TM. Motor axons preferentially reinnervate motor pathways. J Neurosci 1993;13:2730–8.

77. Brushart TM, Gerber J, Kessens P, et al. Contributions of pathway and neuron to preferential motor reinnervation. J Neurosci 1998;18:8674–81.

78. Nix WA, Hopf HC. Electrical stimulation of regenerating nerve and its effect on motor recovery. Brain Res 1983;272:21–5.

79. Al-Majed AA, Brushart TM, Gordon T. Electrical stimulation accelerates and increases expression of BDNF and trkB mRNA in regenerating rat femoral motoneurons. Eur J Neurosci 2000;12:4381–90.

80. Al-Majed AA, Tam SL, Gordon T. Electrical stimulation accelerates and enhances expression of regeneration-associated genes in regenerating rat femoral motoneurons. Cell Mol Neurobiol 2004;24:379–402.

81. Brushart TM, Mesulam MM. Alteration in connections between muscle and anterior horn motoneurons after peripheral nerve repair. Science 1980;208:603–5.

82. Thomas CK, Stein RB, Gordon T, et al. Patterns of reinnervation and motor unit recruitment in human hand muscles after complete ulnar and median nerve section and resuture. J Neurol Neurosurg Psychiatr 1987;50:259–68.

83. Martini R, Schachner M, Brushart TM. The L2/HNK-1 carbohydrate is preferentially expressed by previously motor axon-associated Schwann's cells in reinnervated peripheral nerves. J Neurosci 1994;14:7180–91.

84. Martini R, Xin Y, Schmitz B, et al. The L2/HNK-1 carbohydrate epitope is involved in the preferential outgrowth of motor neurons on ventral roots and motor nerves. Eur J Neurosci 1992;4:628–39.

85. Martini R, Bollensen E, Schachner M. Immunocytological localization of the major peripheral nervous system glycoprotein P0 and the L2/HNK-1 and L3 carbohydrate structures in developing and adult mouse sciatic nerve. Dev Biol 1988;129:330–8.

86. Eberhardt KA, Irintchev A, Al-Majed AA, et al. BDNF/TrkB signaling regulates HNK-1 carbohydrate expression in regenerating motor nerves and promotes functional recovery after peripheral nerve repair. Exp Neurol 2006;198:500–10.

87. Gordon T, Amirjani N, Jones KE, et al. Brief electrical stimulation accelerates axon regeneration and muscle reinnervation in humans. Neuroscience Meeting Planner, Online: Society for Neuroscience; 200. Program No. 872.9/D16.

88. Gordon T, Brushart TM, Amirjani N, et al. The potential of electrical stimulation to promote functional recovery after peripheral nerve injury—comparisons between rats and humans. Acta Neurochir Suppl 2007;100:3–11.

89. Conchello JA, Lichtman JW. Optical sectioning microscopy. Nat Methods 2005;2:920–31.

90. Lichtman JW, Conchello JA. Fluorescence microscopy. Nat Methods 2005;2:910–9.

91. Misgeld T, Kerschensteiner M. In vivo imaging of the diseased nervous system. Nat Rev Neurosci 2006;7:449–63.

92. Helmchen F, Denk W. Deep tissue two-photon microscopy. Nat Methods 2005;2:932–40.

93. Feng G, Mellor RH, Bernstein M, et al. Imaging neuronal subsets in transgenic mice expressing multiple spectral variants of GFP. Neuron 2000;28:41–51.

94. Keller-Peck CR, Walsh MK, Gan WB, et al. Asynchronous synapse elimination in neonatal motor units: studies using GFP transgenic mice. Neuron 2001;31:381–94.

95. Kerschensteiner M, Schwab ME, Lichtman JW, et al. In vivo imaging of axonal degeneration and regeneration in the injured spinal cord. Nat Med 2005;11:572–7.

96. Walsh MK, Lichtman JW. In vivo time-lapse imaging of synaptic takeover associated with naturally occurring synapse elimination. Neuron 2003;37:67–73.

97. Bishop DL, Misgeld T, Walsh MK, et al. Axon branch removal at developing synapses by axosome shedding. Neuron 2004;44:651–61.

98. Zuo Y, Lubischer JL, Kang H, et al. Fluorescent proteins expressed in mouse transgenic lines mark subsets of glia, neurons, macrophages, and dendritic cells for vital examination. J Neurosci 2004;24:10999–1009.

99. Hirrlinger PG, Scheller A, Braun C, et al. Expression of reef coral fluorescent proteins in the central nervous system of transgenic mice. Mol Cell Neurosci 2005;30:291–303.

100. Jung S, Aliberti J, Graemmel P, et al. Analysis of fractalkine receptor CX$_3$CR1 function by targeted deletion and green fluorescent protein reporter gene insertion. Mol Cell Biol 2000;20:4106–14.

101. Misgeld T, Kerschensteiner M, Bareyre FM, et al. Imaging axonal transport of mitochondria in vivo. Nat Methods 2007;4:559–61.

102. Nguyen QT, Sanes JR, Lichtman JW. Pre-existing pathways promote precise projection patterns. Nat Neurosci 2002;5:861–7.

103. Steward O, Zheng B, Tessier-Lavigne M. False resurrections: distinguishing regenerated from spared axons in the injured central nervous system. J Comp Neurol 2003;459:1–8.

104. Baloh RH. Mitochondrial dynamics and peripheral neuropathy. Neuroscientist 2008;14:12–8.

105. Povlishock JT. The fine structure of the axons and growth cones of the human fetal cerebral cortex. Brain Res 1976;114:379.

106. Chada SR, Hollenbeck PJ. Mitochondrial movement and positioning in axons: the role of growth factor signaling. J Exp Biol 2003;206:1985–92.

107. Hollenbeck PJ, Saxton WM. The axonal transport of mitochondria. J Cell Sci 2005;118:5411–9.

108. Pan YA, Misgeld T, Lichtman JW, et al. Effects of neurotoxic and neuroprotective agents on peripheral nerve regeneration assayed by time-lapse imaging in vivo. J Neurosci 2003;23:11479–88.

109. Hayashi A, Koob JW, Liu DZ, et al. A double-transgenic mouse used to track migrating Schwann's cells and regenerating axons following engraftment of injured nerves. Exp Neurol 2007; 207:128–38.

110. Magill CK, Tong A, Kawamura D, et al. Reinnervation of the tibialis anterior following sciatic nerve crush injury: a confocal microscopic study in transgenic mice. Exp Neurol 2007;207:64–74.

Index

Note: Page numbers of article titles are in **boldface** type.

neurosurgery.theclinics.com

Printed and bound by CPI Group (UK) Ltd, Croydon, CR0 4YY

03/10/2024

01040362-0010